And Mother Makes Thirteen

And Mother Makes Thirteen

A Three Sisters Novel of Witchcraft and Betrayal

by

HAROLD L. KLAWANS, M.D.

Author of:
Novels:
SINS OF COMMISSION
INFORMED CONSENT
THE JERUSALEM CODE
DEADLY MEDICINE
CHEKHOV'S LIE

Non-fiction:
TOSCANINI'S FUMBLE
NEWTON'S MADNESS
TRIALS OF AN EXPERT WITNESS
LIFE, DEATH AND IN BETWEEN
WHY MICHAEL COULDN'T HIT

Demos Medical Publishing, Inc., 386 Park Avenue South, New York, New York 10016

Library of Congress Cataloging-in-Publication Data

Klawans, Harold L.
   And mother makes thirteen / Harold L. Klawans.
     p.   cm.
   ISBN 1-888799-20-X
   I. Title.
   PS3561.L336A82   1999   98-55427
   813'.54—dc21   CIP

Made in the United States of America

To my wife Barbara—friend, companion, and muse
And to the other ladies in my life

Debbie

Becky

Emily

Dassi

and

Avi

Prologue

"How were they dressed?" he asked.

"In skirts," Leslie answered hesitantly. Why was therapy still so damn painful for her? Mr. Doran was a good therapist. And he was helping her. She knew that. She did feel more secure. She wasn't frightened anymore and she was sleeping a lot better. Fewer nightmares. No more screaming out in fright. And her grades were improving. Although that course in anthropology was still giving her trouble. Concentrate, she had to concentrate on her therapy. Listen to Mr. Doran. Tell him what he needed to hear. That way he could help her even more. But that was getting harder for her to do. He was probably right. He said that that was part of her progress. She felt better so she didn't want to think about any of it. To remember any of it. But if Mr. Doran was certain that this would help her, she'd do her best. She'd remember all the details. She had to. It was a lot easier than reading Levi-Strauss.

"Leslie."

Leslie thought he sounded almost angry. "Yes," she responded.

"Pay attention. This is for you," he said gently. "So that you can forget it. You can only forget what happened to you by remembering everything. Once you can remember them, none of it will be mysterious. It is only the unknown that is frightening. You have to remember the details."

"I'll try, Mr. Doran. And I know you're right. But sometimes the details aren't that clear. I was so young. I'm not sure I can remember everything. I was only five years old. I. . . ." Her voice trailed off.

"That's why I'm here."

"I know," she responded.

"Leslie. We were talking about the dresses," her therapist reminded her. "The dresses that the women were wearing. The women in your dream."

His voice sounded so soothing. It was relaxing her.

"The dresses." She closed her eyes. The couch was narrow but she was comfortable enough. There was plenty of room for her. She was always comfortable here. She could feel the tension going out of her body. If only she always felt like this. Relaxed. At peace. Not afraid. She was even getting used to the air conditioning. She'd worn a long-sleeved blouse because she knew he'd have the air conditioning on even though it was barely eighty degrees outside. She tried to shut out the whole world when she was here. Her classes. The weather. The rest of her life. Put it all away and climb back into her memory. Into her nightmares.

"The dresses," he repeated softly. "Think about the dresses, Leslie."

She tried. The drone of the air conditioning disappeared, as did the coolness of the leather couch. Then all of a sudden the room was gone. She felt that she was alone. She and Mr. Doran. No. She was all alone. And she wasn't nineteen years old anymore. She wasn't in college.

"The long dresses."

She was back in high school.

"The long black dresses."

In grammar school. The years were being peeled away. Sixth grade. Fourth grade. Third.

"They were long," she began, "very long."

"And they scraped on the ground as they danced. They were dressed completely in black. Remember the dancing. You remembered it before. The dancing. And the dresses."

"I'm getting there. I'm beginning to see them," Leslie said. "They are dancing. And they are dressed in black."

"That's good. Now focus in on them," John Doran instructed her. "Focus on their dresses. The long black dresses, and the dancing. Concentrate. You can remember it all. You were able to remember much of it the last time. They were dancing. The light was flickering. It lit up their faces. In bright colors. Those flames. The orange and yellow flames. Shining on their faces. The dancing faces. On their eyes. Dancing around the. . . ."

"Fire," she said, panting. "We were all dancing around the fire. The bonfire. At the base of the tree."

"What tree?" he asked. She hadn't mentioned the tree before. "Details are very important, Leslie. Tell me what tree it was."

"The tree," she said in a very young voice.

"Which tree?"

Which tree? Her tree. The tree in the backyard. That was the tree. The one with her swing on it. "My tree," she said. "Our tree. The one in our backyard."

"Yes. Your tree. The one in your backyard. And there was a big fire at the base of your tree and they were all dancing around it. How many of them were there?"

Leslie thought hard. She concentrated. She watched them dance. The women. All in black. In the light of the bonfire. She counted them in her mind's eye as they danced in front of her. They were swirling so quickly. Their eyes were so bright. Almost inhuman. And they never blinked. They were almost like reptiles. Eyes of newt. How many of them were there? This was so damn difficult. College was easier. Even anthropology.

"A dozen," she decided. "Twelve." She was proud of herself.

"Count again. Tell me exactly how many there are."

She did ". . . nine, ten, eleven, twelve. A dozen."

"Plus your mother," he told her.

She'd forgotten her. Her own mother. "Plus my mother."

"That makes thirteen. A coven of witches. It's always thirteen. Thirteen is what makes it a coven. That is the magic number. The number with spectral power. That number gives them their demonic strength. Their power."

Mr. Doran was so good. He made her see it all so clearly. Understand it. And it was helping her.

"Think about what happened next," he told her.

She didn't want that. That was what hurt. The blood. The blood in the big bowl. The vessel. It wasn't just any kind of vessel. It was a special type. But she hadn't known what to call it. It was a chalice. The blood-filled chalice.

"Think about the chalice."

She knew what came next. It raced through her mind. The whole scene. As if Mr. Doran had pushed the fast forward button. But the witches were still there and they were still dancing. Their eyes were still staring at her. And the fire was still burning bright. And the flames. She counted them again.

Twelve. There were only twelve of them. Her mother. Where was her mother? "My mom, I don't see my mom. She's not dancing anymore. The others still are. She isn't. There are only twelve witches dancing around me." Her voice was harsh now and frightened.

"She has to be there. Concentrate."

She was. Her mother had to be there. Not dancing around her but with her. Holding her. Her mother was holding her. Holding her mouth open. Pouring in the blood.

Making her swallow the blood.

And then not letting her up.

Holding her.

Helping him yank off her clothes. Her dress. Her panties.

Holding her. Forcing her. Her knees. Her legs. Her. . . .

Forcing her. Them. Apart.

For him.

For her father.

For her father to. . . .

Under the tree.

Under her own tree. He did it to her under her tree. Below her own swing. Her own father. Thank God he was dead. Thank God. . . . Her father. . . . She screamed. "It wasn't my father," she said softly. "It was that . . . that . . ."she was now sobbing softly.

"Wasn't your father?"

"It couldn't have been. Not my real father."

"It had to be. Who else could. . . ?"

"No. No." She was crying now.

"But it happened. You were . . . violated."

"I was . . . raped," she sobbed. "But it wasn't my father. It couldn't have been."

"Your mother? Wasn't she there?"

"She was there."

"She held you."

"Yes."

"So, it was your father."

"No, it was my stepfather."

"Your stepfather? How can you be sure?"

"The tree."

"Your tree?"

"My tree. It wasn't my tree. It was his tree. It was his house. We moved into that house when my mom married him." She was crying harder. Not out of pain. Or fear. Or sadness. But out of a peculiar mixture of emotions. "I'll get that son of a bitch."

"Your stepfather? I never. . . ."

Chapter
1

Dennie Cater paid the cabdriver and shoved her wallet back into her purse before she even attempted to open the back door of the cab. God, she hated the cruelty of February in Chicago. And the wind. Especially the wind. Her first attempt was only partially successful. As soon as she pried the door partially open, the harsh winter wind tearing off Lake Michigan blew it shut. The second time she wedged it open with her shoulder and then worked her way out of the back seat. We like the change of seasons, she reminded herself. That's why we live in Chicago. Because we like to tell that lie to each other. The windchill, she was certain, was at least forty below. Once she was out of the cab, the wind slammed the door shut behind her and threw her toward the doorway of the skyscraper that loomed up in front of her, crashing her into the revolving door, which spun her into the building. Once inside, she crossed the lobby to the back bank of elevators, entered the waiting car, and pushed the button for the seventy-second floor. That was the home of Keneally and Keneally, one of Chicago's more powerful law firms. Only then did the chill begin to depart. To hell with the change of seasons.

Dennie liked Sean Keneally. She'd liked him when she first met him and that hadn't changed over the last five years. Sean was as Irish as his name. The family had been in Chicago for three generations. Long enough to have the right connections in a city where the right connections still counted. Dennie had also grown up well connected so she easily accepted his clout. And Sean never flaunted it. She liked working for him. Not only did his firm pay well, they also paid promptly. Not all law firms did that. Defense firms often merely forwarded their bills on to the insurance companies, which got around to paying them three months later. That was, she had learned, what the insurance business was all about. Her older sister, Jessie, had taught her that. Jessie was the numbers person in the family. Insurance companies got their money upfront and held onto it for as long as possible. That was because most of their income came from the interest they collected on the money they held, so they always paid as late as they possibly could. Or a couple of months later. And the plaintiff firms were always waiting for the

1

next settlement. They all worked on consignment. They got a percentage of the settlement.

The door finally closed and the elevator started to move. Her teeth chattered one more time. One more shiver shook her shoulders. Dennie didn't work on consignment. She would never get rich if a client got a big judgment. She always worked on a straight fee for time basis. Not fee for service. Not fee for results. And there was no tipping. Fee for time. Forty dollars per hour per investigator. Except that she and two of her sisters were not licensed investigators. If someone needed a label for what they did, they supplied one. They called themselves paralegals. Three Sisters Limited, Paralegals to the World. To the world of small law firms that needed somebody with their experience and talents only part-time and to large firms like Keneally and Keneally when they needed something done quickly and quietly and in a way that would be very hard to trace back to them. Clout liked secrecy.

The door opened. She could feel the opulence. She had to be on the right floor.

Should she raise their fee? From forty to fifty bucks an hour? Keneally and Keneally could afford it. So could their clients. Any client who could afford Sean could pay another ten bucks an hour. Hell, they wouldn't even feel it. Or notice it. She'd already put in six hours. Keneally and Keneally occupied the entire seventy-second floor. There was a reception desk opposite the elevators. The receptionist smiled at her. The smile seemed to be a permanent fixture, like the silk flowers. Only slightly less perishable.

"Dennie Cater," she said, identifying herself.

"Mr. Keneally is waiting for you in the conference room. It's. . . ."

"Just where it used to be, I suppose," Dennie cut her off.

The receptionist's smile seemed to skip a beat.

"I'll find it myself," Dennie said, with a very broad smile of her own, almost a grin. She turned and walked down the wide hall, past the large Paschke oil painting of a flickering TV screen with its images not quite in focus, but none the less vivid. She loved that picture. Sean had bought it after the Paschke show had returned from its stay at the Pompidou in Paris. It would never have been his father's choice. His father never advanced beyond Monet. No, he never got as far as Monet. He barely got to Renoir. And Degas. All those pretty little girls without too many clothes. Certainly not Cézanne.

The doors of the conference room were open. The room had to be at least twenty by thirty-five; with thirty-five feet of thick plate glass window looking northward out over the rooftops of the city. Toward North Lake Shore Drive. And Navy Pier. And the beaches and the lagoons, and the yacht harbors, and the deserted lake itself. Lake Michigan. She loved that view even on a drab February day with no boats in sight. The water was a dark, choppy gray. And it would become a deep blue in just a couple of months. God, she loved the change of seasons. Now that she was no longer cold. It wasn't February that was all that cruel.

Sean was staring out the window. He was forty-two. He'd turned forty-two on January 22nd. He kept himself in great shape. Six one. One sixty five. And not an ounce of fat. And just enough gray hair to look distinguished. And so damn trustworthy. Fatherly. As if that were a guarantee of trustworthiness. Hadn't Stalin been someone's father? Or Machiavelli? And what about Attila? Her teeth chattered again. More like a battery of tympani than a mere drumroll. Another series of shivers ran through her. February! Dennie wondered if he added that gray. He'd had those streaks of gray five years ago when he and Jessie had first become lovers. She'd have to ask Jessie. Jessie would know. She'd ask Jessie. When she comes back to work. When. . . .

"Denise," he said, turning away from the view.

He was the only man she let call her Denise. It was the only name Sean ever used. They'd met through Jessie. Right after the two of them had split up. Why hadn't it worked out for the two of them? She thought she knew why but she wasn't certain. And that she could not ask Jessie. Now or when she came home. Or ever. Had Jessie thought of him as a father figure? Older? Secure? Stable? Comforting? The chill just wouldn't leave her body.

"Sean," she replied.

"Sit," he nodded, leaving all the rest unsaid.

She sat at one end of the broad mahogany table. The painting behind her was by another of Chicago's imagists, Roger Brown. She had not seen it before, but she recognized the style immediately. It was a map of the United States covered by a myriad of strip malls. Brown's vision of the future of an America paved by strip malls, K-Marts from coast to coast. Or were they Wal-Marts? Did it matter? Except to the stockholders? It was a future that had already arrived. The table had a highly polished finish. She could see the reflection of her own face. And of her blond hair. It needed to be trimmed. If not hacked off.

Sean sat down at the other end of the table, just over twenty feet away. His face was friendly, thin but not harsh. He had the nicest smile. No wonder clients trusted him. No wonder Jessie had. Behind him was a large painting of Comiskey Park. Why did men love baseball so? Because it gave them a chance to play with their bats and balls. In public. No. Then women should also love it. And she hated it. "I've done some background work," she said.

"Good."

"Eight hours," she said. "But those are only my hours. Elizabeth put in a lot of time too," she quickly added.

He waved her off with an ever so slight shake of his head, like a pitcher waving off a sign. She smiled at her metaphor. Or was it a simile? Beth had been the English major. That seemed a lifetime ago. When they were undergraduates. "Just send a bill. And it's still sixty an hour, isn't it?"

She nodded, almost as imperceptibly. Two could play that game. And they could use the money. Jessie's treatment was taking far longer than they had expected. God, she missed her.

"I checked him out pretty thoroughly," she began.

"Dr. Doran," he nodded.

"He's not a doctor."

"I know. He's not a physician," Sean replied. "He's some sort of other kind of doctor."

"He's not a doctor of any sort. Not an M.D. Not a Ph.D. Not any kind of a 'D' at all. No doctorate degree. Just a master's degree. In clinical psychology. And he doesn't claim to be a doctor either. Not on his cards. Nor his stationery. Nor his ads in *The Reader.*

"Dr. Doran advertises in *The Reader?*"

"Mr. Doran," she reminded him.

"Mr. Doran, I stand corrected," Sean smiled.

It truly was a great smile. Full of warmth. Comfort. Reassuring. Her body began to relax. The edge was off the chill. "At least he went to a real school," she continued.

"Where?"

"U. of I.," she informed him. "At Champaign-Urbana. He got his bachelor's in '58 and his master's in '60. And he's been in private practice as a counselor ever since."

"But he doesn't have a doctorate; so he's not a real therapist."

"And I'm not a real investigator," she reminded him.

"Touché."

"And he's pretty clean as far as I can tell. He's got no police record. There have never been any complaints to the cops about him. No lawsuits. Past or present. He lives pretty modestly. Well within his income. He drives a six year old Maxima. Has a wife. Two grown kids. No lovers as far as anyone knows. Of either sex."

"So he doesn't cheat on his wife or his patients?"

"Probably not," she conceded carefully.

"You sound skeptical. Tell me about those ads. The ones in *The Reader.* What's he advertise for?"

"Women. Young women."

"Young women! Why?"

"That's who he specializes in treating. Young women. College girls mostly. With trouble hacking it. Except it's called situational stress in his parlance. Or acute adjustment reactions. Or depression."

"Just young women," Sean pondered his own statement.

"Not exclusively young women, but mostly. And mostly young women with good insurance. Or well-to-do fathers."

"Of course. I understand his predilection for patients with good insurance, but why just women? Is he into young women? Something kinky? Or. . . ."

Dennie did not reply at first.

"Denise, spill it."

"He has a ceiling made of glass."

"What?"

"A ceiling made of glass. That's a line from a song by Rodgers and Hart. A ceiling made of glass."

"Where?"

"In his office," she replied. "Where else? I went there. I played the confused yuppie. Needing some help. I have all the right credentials. I'm young enough to be in graduate school. I have great insurance."

"And your dad was very rich."

"At one time."

He said nothing. There was no reason to confirm the truth.

"So I went to his office carrying my ad from *The Reader*. It was all on the up and up. As far as I could tell. He sat at his desk. I sat opposite him. Nothing funny. I talked about my screwed up social life."

"Is it?"

"That's none of your business. Nor his. I tried hard to make sure that nothing I told him had any semblance of truth in it. He listened for a few minutes. And told me that my relationships with the men in my life were not the problem but were merely a symptom of a deeper problem and that working on that would take time. I asked him to explain. And he did. All the usual mumbo jumbo. Freud, Adler, Jung. You name it. And while he did that I looked around his office. At his degrees. U. of I. Some postgraduate courses in therapy some-place in Florida. And a couple of certificates from the Jung Institute here in Chicago. And all the right books. The complete works of Freud. And of Jung. And then I saw it."

"What?"

"The ceiling of glass," she reminded him.

"Where?"

"Above the couch."

"What is it? Some sort of mirror to look at while he's screwing his patients?"

"You have an adolescent imagination."

"Is that what Jessica told you?"

"No. She never complained about your . . . ah . . . imagination."

"So what is it?"

"Worse. Or maybe better."

"Better? How could it be better?"

"It's about one foot by one foot. And it's not a mirror to look at. It's to look through. To film through. I figure he takes videotapes of all his sessions."

"Why does he do that?"

"I could come up with two reasons. One may be just to protect himself. If he ever gets sued, he has tapes of what really happened. After all, he treats a lot of young women. Young women with problems. If they didn't have problems, he wouldn't be treating them. And patients often have fantasies. Fantasies about their therapists."

"That sounds like a potentially dangerous combination," Sean admitted. "Very potent, no pun intended."

"None perceived. I figure he might tape his interviews for self-protection."

"But why video? Audio is cheaper and would be just as much protection. He could be like Richard Nixon."

"Video is better for the second reason."

"What's that?"

"Training. He's a student at the Institute for Jungian Analysis and he may relive those sessions with one of the training analysts. Videotaping lets them both see precisely what happened. Both verbally and nonverbally. That way they can analyze everything together."

"So he's clean?"

"Unless he screws only some of his patients and watches the films himself later."

"Is that what you think he does."

"No," she didn't. "But he could. He certainly has the temptation and the opportunity."

"Too bad."

"Why too bad? Your client is one of his patients."

"Yes, but if we had something on him, then he might be more willing to testify for her. So many therapists hate going to court. They figure they just get caught in the middle. Their job is to help their patients emotionally. Not in court."

"They may be right about that."

"But I need his help to get that SOB."

Dennie nodded. "I'm going to look at some of his tapes."

"How. . . ? No, don't tell me. I don't want to know."

The phone buzzed. His client had arrived. A few moments later Ms. Smiles opened the door and showed the client in. Leslie English looked very small in her long black leather coat. She stood in the doorway as if she were not quite certain where she should go or what she should do or say. Sean knew just what to do. He moved quickly to the doorway and gave her a fatherly hug. A chill cut through Dennie. Leslie had brought winter into the room with her. The younger woman did not hug him back but neither did she freeze or pull away. That, Dennie assumed, was a very good sign. All things considered, fatherly affection might not be one of the things she accepted readily. Sean kept his arm on her shoulder and escorted her to his end of the mahogany table. He helped her take off her coat and then folded it over the back of one of the empty leather chairs. Her coat and the chairs made a good match. Only an expert could tell which leather was more expensive.

Leslie sat down in the chair next to the coat. She was two chairs away from the father figure. Not too close for comfort. The chair seemed to dwarf her. She had not once looked at the art. Or the view out the window. So much for the dramatic view of ice-covered Lake Michigan. And the expensive decor.

Sean sat back in his chair and introduced the two women. They both already knew some details about each other. Sean didn't have to supply any preliminary explanations.

Dennie had requested the meeting. She had hoped it would save her time. It was up to her to get things started.

"Tell me," Dennie began, "why did you go to see John Doran in the first place?"

Leslie did not look at her, but looked down at her fingernails as if her manicure needed checking. "Do you want to know why I needed to see a therapist? Or why I chose to see John Doran?"

"Or both?" Dennie added, wondering at the source of Leslie's hostility. Dennie wanted to help her.

Leslie looked at Dennie for the first time. "Or both?"

"Both."

"Mr. Doran had helped a friend of mine. She was having a problem with . . . with . . . ," Leslie stopped.

"Yes," promptly. Leslie's selection of Mr. Doran had not been a random response to an advertisement. He had been recommended by a friend. "And . . ." Dennie prompted the younger woman once again.

"A problem . . . ah . . . one of her professors was putting the make on her. It was getting pretty intense."

"And Mr. Doran helped her?"

"Yes."

"Why didn't she just go to the dean?" Dennie asked.

Leslie was once again looking at her nails.

"That was sexual harassment of a student. That could cost him his job. You don't need a therapist to take care of that," Dennie reminded her. "Most schools are pretty sensitive to that sort of stuff. He would have had the problem."

"It wasn't that simple."

˜ Perhaps the professor had a ceiling of glass. Perhaps something had happened before the friend wanted it to stop. Perhaps. . . ."I'm listening," Dennie said.

"He. . . ."

"Yes. He. . . ."

"Was a she. And the problem was that my friend wasn't sure whether. . . . They're now living together."

"Your friend and the professor?"

"Yes."

"And Mr. Doran helped her?"

"Yes, he helped her. He helped her sort out her real feelings. It wasn't the professor she wanted to reject. It was her parents. It. . . ." Leslie stopped on her own.

It all sounded so familiar. But that was what made Freud universal. We all spend our lives reliving the past. It's only a matter of emphasis. "And she thought Doran could help you?"

"Yes."

Leslie was not entirely the lost little waif she appeared to be. "Why?"

"I was raped," Leslie informed her tersely

"By your own stepfather," Dennie spit out through clenched teeth, surprised at the level of anger in her own voice.

"No. By my roommate's brother. On a date." She said it coldly, matter-of-factly, without emotion. "Last spring. It was on our second date. We'd gone out to dinner. Then to see a movie. Then he took me back to my apartment. He came up to see his sister. She was out. So he . . . he. . . . I couldn't tell anyone. First I was worried I was pregnant. He hadn't used anything. And I use a diaphragm. I couldn't. He wouldn't. . . . And he didn't. . . . Then I was scared that I had VD or something. Then I was just angry. Seething. Mad at him. And his sister. And myself. At the whole damn world. I blew off my finals. My life wasn't worth a shit. I . . . I. . . . Then this friend told me about Mr. Doran and how great a therapist he was, so I went to see him. What the hell. Things could- n't have gotten much worse."

"And?"

"He helped me."

"How?"

"He made me understand my feelings. What had really happened to me. What I was really responding to. My real anger. I wasn't mad at Peter. It was . . . I mean

I was mad at Peter. I liked him but I didn't want to sleep with him. Not yet. Not then. Not like that. But I didn't stop him. Why couldn't I? Why didn't I? He helped me remember. It wasn't Peter who raped me. He did. I know that. But I let him because . . . because. . . ."

"Your stepfather had already done it to you. More than. . . ." Control your anger, Dennie reminded herself. "And you were just reliving that rape with Peter. And since you couldn't stop your stepfather, you couldn't stop Peter."

"Yes. My stepfather. That dirty bastard."

"And now you are suing that bastard."

"You're damn right I am."

"And Ms. Cater is going to help you," Sean chimed in.

They were both startled by Sean Keneally's intrusion into their private conversation.

"How?" the younger woman asked.

"Two ways," Dennie replied. "First we need some real evidence of all that witchcraft business. We're going to work on that and my sister is also working on Mr. Doran."

"Mr. Doran? He's my therapist. I'm not sure. . . ."

"Like all therapists, he'd rather not be involved," Sean commented. "And we need his help. His testimony."

"So what is your sister going to do?" Leslie asked, looking straight at Dennie Cater.

"Make sure he wants to be involved."

"How will she do that?"

"Don't worry. That's her problem," Dennie informed her.

"How?" Leslie asked again.

"Did you know that he makes tapes of all his sessions?"

"Tapes?"

Either she didn't know or she was a good actress. Or, Dennie reminded herself, both. "He makes videotapes of all his sessions."

"Wow! You're kidding."

She doubted that Leslie was that good an actress. That meant that she didn't know. Did any of his other patients? Leslie's friend probably didn't. She hadn't warned Leslie. Such knowledge might not be good for business. "No, I'm not kidding."

"But how will that help me?"

"I'm not sure it will," Dennie admitted.

"Wow, tapes. That's creepy."

"Could there be anything on those tapes that might help us?" she asked Leslie.

"Like something with one of his patients?"

"Like something like that."

"Kinky."

"Was there anything kinky with you?"

"And Mr. Doran? Never."

The three of them spent the next half hour going over every detail that Leslie could remember about what her stepfather had done to her and how often and exactly what she'd told Doran. This was very different from her sessions with Mr. Doran. No one was helping her. They were just firing questions. One after another. Firing and cross-firing. Almost as if they were preparing her for trial. Which, in a way, they were.

When they were done, they were all tired. And the process had not added much to what Sean had already told Dennie. Leslie's memories were all fuzzy at best. It was unclear how many times it had happened. Once. Twice. Three times. Habitually. Was that why there were no specific details? No specific memories chiseled into stone? Not the recall of a single event, but of an ongoing process. Over time.

And over what time frame? Days? Weeks? Months? Years? When had it started? When had it stopped? One fact was clear. There were other witnesses to at least one of the incidents. What a euphemism. To one of the rapes. To the first rape. The ritual rape. There had been witnesses. Twelve of them. Those other witches. The rest of the coven. They had been there. They had seen what had been done to her. Leslie gave them the names she could remember. She could only be certain of three names. She might have remembered more during therapy. She'd given those names to Mr. Doran. Dennie could get them from him. They'd be on her videotape.

"And your mother," Dennie reminded them all.

"Yes, my mother."

"Hopefully we can leave her out of this," Sean said.

"For Leslie's sake?" Dennie asked.

"No. For the case. It'll be better if it's just her stepfather."

Dennie understood. It was time for her to go. She got up to leave.

"Make sure Elizabeth behaves herself," Sean reminded Dennie.

"I will. And she will. It'll all be usable in court. Good clean evidence. Well documented. As good as the FBI."

"Let's hope so. And give my love to Jessica."

"I'll do that when I talk to her."

❋❋❋❋

The cab dropped Dennie off in front of her apartment building, just south of downtown. Her teeth were hardly chattering. As long as she didn't think about

Leslie she could control them. Easier thought than done. Not even a muffled drumroll. The wind had died down. She had no trouble opening the door of the cab. She and Beth had lived there for seven years, ever since the building had been rehabed. It had once been an industrial property, a print factory of some sort in a neighborhood of old printing shops. That was what it was called now. Not just their building, but the whole region. Printer's Row. Dennie loved this building with its high ceilings. And thick walls. And even thicker ceilings. All nice and private. She even liked the ceilings without any glass on them. She chuckled bitterly to herself. She picked up their mail. There were no checks. No bills. A few pieces of junk mail. That made it a good day. They had broken even. No cash flow at all. Then she walked up the one long flight of stairs to their floor. She never took the elevator. Not for the exercise. Beth was the one sister who was into exercise. Dennie ran from time to time. Often more to work out some anxiety. She loved the old woodwork on the stairway. Oak. Almost as rich as the table in Sean's conference room.

Her answering machine was flashing. As she slipped off her coat, Dennie pushed the button. The machine whirred and then began to play.

"Hi," the message began. "It's me. Beth. I'm just checking in. Quiet day. I'll pay Doran's office a visit tonight. Don't worry. I'll be very careful. His receptionist is a doll. But very stupid. I'll have no trouble getting in. Talk to you later."

Dennie heard the telltale click and then a beep. "It's Friday. Four forty-four P.M.," the computer voice added.

"Hi," another voice began. "It's me. Jessie." Dennie smiled. They'd both checked in. "Just called to tell you I'm fine. I'm glad you're working with Sean. He's a good guy. And it never hurts to have political connections. Not in Chicago. And he pays well. Give him my love. I'll be home soon."

Click. Beep. "It's Friday. Four forty-eight P.M."

Beep. Beep. Beep. There were no more messages.

And it was still Friday. Just a few minutes after five. She'd stay home, have a quiet dinner by herself, read a good book, and be there in case Beth called and needed some help.

✳✳✳✳

It was six o'clock. She looked at her treadmill and rolled over. Ten more minutes, she thought to herself. Ten more minutes. Then the phone rang. She grabbed it.

"Beth," she assumed.

"Denise," a male voice said.

"Who is this?"

"Sean, Sean Keneally. Who is this?"

"Dennie. You did call me."

"Denise, I know I called you. Is Elizabeth home yet?"

"I . . . I don't know. She wasn't home when I went to bed and she didn't wake me up. She usually doesn't. Why?"

"Somebody killed John Doran and the police seem to think Elizabeth might have done it."

"She couldn't have. Not Beth. She wouldn't hurt a flea."

"Neither of us believes that," Sean contradicted her.

"Perhaps not." It was the strongest argument she could muster on such short notice. It was a good thing she wasn't a lawyer.

"And he wasn't a flea. He was a man with a video camera and a ceiling made of glass."

"You don't believe. . . . "

"Just thought I'd warn you both."

"Thanks."

"The cops should be there any minute." Jessie was right about one thing. In this town political connections never hurt.

Suddenly someone was pounding on the front door.

"It's the police," a voice announced.

"They're here," she told Sean. His warning had come just in the nick of time. Or had it? Beth! Where was she?

Chapter II

"Just a minute," Dennie called out. She pulled on her thin silken robe and went into the kitchen. The two apartments were connected by a small doorway that they had had built into their kitchens. That was the one advantage to owning their own apartments. They were able to make such alterations. As always, the door was closed, but not locked. There was no lock. They'd never seen a need for a lock. They respected each other's privacy. And the only time Beth had walked in on someone unannounced, he was the one who was embarrassed. Dennie had already gone to work. And so should he have. Making toast without bothering to put his clothes on. It served him right.

She heard her doorbell ring again, as she scampered into Beth's kitchen and then she crossed into her sister's bedroom. Beth was not there. Dennie would have bet that she wouldn't be. She'd just had to make certain. Beth was not always reliable. The bed looked like it hadn't been slept in for weeks. It probably hadn't. Whenever Beth fell in love that seemed to happen. Dennie shrugged her shoulders and dashed into Beth's living room. Beth's typewriter was there, but she hadn't left any messages in it. It was one of her favorite means of communication. That's what their mother had often done. Leave messages typed in her typewriter for her little girls. If only Beth would learn to use something less archaic. Even a dedicated word processor. Then she could send messages directly onto Dennie's machine. No need to intrude. No chance of embarrassing anyone. But not Beth. If it was good enough for mom. . . . Next to the typewriter Dennie found just what she was looking for. Beth's appointment book and her matching address book. Dennie grabbed them both and raced back into her kitchen. The doorbell was ringing once again. Still. Where should she put the diary? And the address book? On her own desk. Where else would they belong? She then threw her own into the bottom desk drawer. They looked as if they belonged. A nice leather desk set. That done, she then walked into the front bathroom, flushed the toilet, and yelled, "Hold your horses."

Dennie then counted to ten and walked to her front door and looked out through the small peephole. A man was standing there with his hands in the pockets of his black leather jacket. He was impatiently shifting his weight from

13

foot to foot. Obviously the source of the urgency. He looked to be about forty, maybe a couple of years older. Six foot one or two. He wore no hat. No muffler. And his coat was unbuttoned, even though it was six o'clock on a cold February morning. Probably thought it was more macho that way. She'd guess that he weighed one eighty. Maybe a bit more. The coat was rather bulky. He wore woolen trousers. And his shoes were of good quality leather.

His face was only slightly weathered. And his eyes were dark but otherwise hard to read in the dimly lit hallway. He was again reaching for the bell. "Show me some ID," she said through the closed door.

The man reached inside his coat with his left hand and pulled out a leather folder, which he flipped open to reveal a badge. It was a badge. Was it real? How the hell was she supposed to know? She'd never seen a real Chicago police badge up close. Only crooks would have enough experience to know the difference. But it was what you were supposed to do.

"Ms. Cater?" the man said, still holding his badge up to the buttonhole. He certainly wasn't trying to hide it or pocket it quickly.

"You probably got that at some hockshop," she called out as she opened the door. It wasn't so much that the badge convinced her, but she was expecting the police. She stood in the open doorway staring at the man.

"Ward," he said. "Lieutenant Tom Ward. I'm from Homicide." That, too, did not surprise her. He was staring back at her at least as intently as she was staring at him. And his stare was more intense. He was undoubtedly better at this game. Probably part of his training.

She felt the chill of the cold air swirling in from the hallway and cutting through her white silken robe. God, she hated that feeling. It was like yesterday only worse. She should have put on something heavier. And thicker. She did have a terrycloth robe. Why had she grabbed this one?

"Ms. Cater?" he said once again.

"Yes," she said, not asking him in.

He was still staring directly at her. Why? Did she look that peculiar? Her hair, she knew, was disheveled. It had that just slept in look. Very appropriate for someone who had just been awakened from a sound sleep. And she was certain her eyes had bags under them. Even more appropriate, since her sleep had not been that sound. His eyes. In the half-dark of the hallway, she couldn't even be sure of their color. The only good illumination was coming from behind her.

Behind her! So that was why he was staring. She should have put on something darker. And less transparent. No, less translucent. She was glad she'd remembered the right word. Beth would be proud of her. At least she should have pulled on some underwear. That she wished very much, but right now she had had more important things to do. "Well," she demanded.

"You have the right to remain silent. . . . " he began.

"The right. What the hell is this?"

"I'm reading you your rights."

"What am I suspected of? Indecent exposure?"

"No. Nothing is indecent. And nothing is exposed as far as I can tell," he said, almost apologetically.

"So?"

"Suspicion of murder. But we both know that."

"Of whom?" As if she didn't know.

"John Doran, as if you don't know."

Dennie nodded. It was obvious to both of them that she was not surprised by this news. "So why are you standing in the hall staring at me?" she asked.

"I'm waiting for my partner to get here with the warrant."

"And you are staring because you figure if you look hard enough, I won't disappear. Or is it that you just like the view?"

"I might like the view if I could really see it," he explained. "It's these new soft contacts. I just got them today. I was fitted last week. But I picked 'em up yesterday afternoon. This is the first time I've worn them. And I've had them in for ten hours now and they're killing me. Can I come in and use your bathroom? It won't count as if you asked me in. I'll come back out here. I promise."

"Okay with me," she said, stepping back.

While he used her front bathroom, Dennie ducked into her closet and pulled on a pair of sweat pants and a sweat shirt that didn't quite match. They met just outside the bathroom. He now had on a pair of glasses. Horn-rimmed glasses. His eyes, she could see, were a deep blue. Yet soft. And he looked younger. And stronger. And. . . .

"Thanks," he said. "I'll wait in the hall, Ms. Cater. I think my partner will be here with the warrant in a few minutes."

He walked across her front room, "Thanks again, Elizabeth," he said.

"I can't accept your thanks."

"Because I'm about to arrest you?"

"No, because my name isn't Elizabeth."

"Isn't Elizabeth? Your name is Cater. That's what it says on your door. I could see that much."

He wasn't the first person who had made that mistake. "It says Cater, all right. But that's not for Elizabeth Cater. It's for Denise. Denise Cater. Most people call me Dennie. Elizabeth is my sister. Everyone calls her Beth. She lives next door."

"There's no name on that doorway," he remarked, as if that were somehow new information.

"She likes her privacy."

"Sorry I bothered you, Ms. Cater. Do you know if the other Ms. Cater is at home?"

Did she? "No."

"No, she's not at home?"

"No. No, I don't know whether she's at home or not. I'm not my sister's keeper. Look, Lieutenant. . . . "

"Tom," he interrupted.

She ignored his intrusion. "Why don't you sit down and relax your eyes some more. I'll run next door and check."

"Okay," he said, walking over to her leather couch and sitting down. "Nice paintings," he added.

"I don't think of them as nice," she said. "Reproductions of Van Gogh are nice." She was sorry she said that. It had been a knee-jerk reaction. She loved the art she collected. It was all strong. And vibrant. By Chicago imagist painters. *Nice* was not the right word.

"You're right," he apologized, with a smile. It was a nice smile. Very genuine. "I grew up down the street from the Paschkes. That's a good Paschke. Done around seventy-two, wasn't it?"

"Yes." Why was this man a cop? He didn't fit her stereotype of cops. Not because he grew up near Ed Paschke. One Polish neighborhood wasn't that different from any other, but he knew Paschke's work well enough to date it. And date it correctly.

"I collect Wirsum myself. They're a lot cheaper. Not any less original. Not any less inventive. Just cheaper. And on my salary, that's important, and besides, I need the humor. In my line of work, I need all the humor I can get."

"That may be why he's cheaper."

"The humor?"

"Yes. Critics all look down at humor. They love Eugene O'Neill and sniff at Kaufman and Hart. And poor Neil Simon. Humor is almost as disreputable as writing murder mysteries."

"And look, I apologize. I really wasn't staring at you. I wouldn't do that. Not that I wouldn't like what I'd see. I would. Very much, I think. But . . . you know. . . . I. . . ."

"Apology accepted," she said. "Be back in a minute."

She walked down the hallway into her kitchen and crossed into Beth's apartment. The two apartments were twins. No, mirror images. There was a scientific word for that. Beth knew it. She always knew the right word. Maybe not the right thing to do, but always the right word for whatever she was doing. What was that word? The two apartments were like identical twins except that

Beth's kitchen had been converted into a large walk-in pantry. Beth hated to cook. So she had no need for a kitchen. All she ever made was coffee.

Dennie walked into Beth's bedroom. Was there anything else that had to be confiscated? To be kept out of Tom Ward's eyesight? There was. Mike's picture. Where was it? Mike was a cop. What Beth saw in a cop, Dennie never knew. Maybe Mike liked Paschke, too. Or Roger Brown. Or Karl Wirsum. She doubted it. Beth didn't. She was into Georgia O'Keeffe. Especially O'Keeffe's flowers. She had reproductions of them all over the walls.

Mike's picture was on Beth's bedside table, in one of those cardboard standup folders. Dennie grabbed it and shoved it under her sweat shirt, half inside her sweat pants. She surveyed the bedroom. There was nothing else that had to be removed. The bed. Should she muss it? Shouldn't she? She debated. She decided not to. Next came the bathroom. Okay. The living room. Nothing.

She walked quickly back into her own living room. Tom Ward was not where she had left him. He was sitting at her desk, his elbows on the desk, his hands cradling his forehead. The leather desk set was all but jumping out at him and yelling "read me." But his eyes were closed.

"Tom," she said, "you okay?"

"My eyes still hurt," he said. "The things we do for vanity."

"She's not home," Dennie told him.

"Somehow I didn't think she would be." He sat back, and the chair leaned back fifteen or twenty degrees. He swiveled it to the right. "Tell me about the picture."

"Which one?" she asked, startled by his question.

"The mannequin out of a Frederick's of Hollywood catalog," he said, pointing to the picture he was describing, of a female form bedecked in complex and yet somehow threatening undergarments.

Perhaps he didn't know as much about Chicago art as she thought. "It's by Ramberg. Christina Ramberg." Ramberg was one of the original imagists. Anyone who was into Chicago art. . . .

"Damn it, I couldn't remember her name. I saw her retrospective at the Renaissance Society. It's a great picture."

"Beth gave it to me for my birthday last year."

"Tell me about her."

"She's quite ill. Mentally. Neurologically, I mean. She's got Pick's disease. That's like Alzheimer's, only worse."

"Your sister?"

"I thought you meant Christina Ramberg."

He swung the chair around so that he was now facing her and the desk. And the leather diary and address book. Mike's address was in that book. And God knows what was in the diary. The fun and games were over. No more sparring. No more art appreciation. His eyes looked much harder now. So did his entire face. "Tell me about your sister."

"I have two sisters," she began.

"No more games."

"I'm not playing a game, but the best way to tell you about Beth is to tell you all about the three of us. We're very close. All three of us."

He nodded.

"Can I sit down?" Why had she asked that? This was her home. He was a guest in her house.

"Why are you asking me that?" he asked her. "This is your home. I'm a guest in your house."

She ambled over to the leather chair beneath the Christina Ramberg. That image ought to be enough to keep him from staring at her.

The lieutenant never even turned the chair to face her. Instead he merely leaned back and looked up at the ceiling. She couldn't tell if his eyes were open or closed. "Tell me about all three of the sisters."

They had, she began, always been very close. It was a story she had told so often before that it almost came out without thinking. There was less than two years separating the three of them. Twenty-three months was all. "Jessica's the oldest. Most people call her Jessie. Then comes me, Denise AKA Dennie. And Elizabeth is the youngest."

"Known as Beth?"

"Usually. We grew up in the western suburbs. Dan Cater was our father."

"Of D. Cater Construction."

"None other. But you must already know that much."

"I do. Your dad had more political ties than Warhol painted soup cans."

There was no reason for her to make any comment at all. They both knew that he was right. And his correctness needed no confirmation. It was a fact. Like the roundness of the world.

"Your brother runs the firm now."

Another fact not in need of any sort of confirmation. Merely modification.

"Half brother . . . David."

"Half. . . ?"

"His mother was killed when he was five. Then dad got remarried, to our Mom. David was part of the deal."

"Killed?"

"A freak accident of some sort. I don't know what. I'm not sure I ever did. He was just our older brother. He must be almost forty now."

"And you?"

What did that matter? Not exactly relevant to whatever he was investigating. "We're twenty-eight."

"All three of you?"

"Yes."

"How can you all be the same age?"

"We can't. But we decided long ago that we'd all go by my age. We were almost like triplets."

"No oldest sister that way."

"And no baby sister either."

They grew up like all kids do. And went their separate ways for a while. They went to different colleges.

"Mom died when we were in college. A heart attack. She'd been diabetic all her life. Insulin-dependent. Jessie's a numbers person. A degree in accounting— then an MBA. All that kind of thing. Dad had been grooming her to be the comptroller of the company. Beth was an English major. Then went for a graduate degree in comparative literature. Russian literature. Chekhov. All that stuff."

"And you?"

"Nothing special. I majored in psychology. The world's most useless degree. Then I trained to be a paralegal."

"Why not law school?"

"I was considering that. But then dad got sick. Acute leukemia. So he set up this firm for the three of us."

"Three Sisters Limited."

"Yes. The idea for the name was Beth's."

He nodded.

"From Chekhov," she explained.

"I didn't think it was from *Macbeth*."

"Touché." An educated cop.

"And what exactly does Three Sisters Limited do?" he asked. It was perhaps his first pertinent inquiry.

"Paralegal work."

"Meaning what, exactly? That's a euphemism that could cover a lot of sins."

"Not too many sins. Mostly we work with law firms who need help in our areas of expertise."

"Which are?"

"White-collar crime."

"Why do three heiresses like you have to work for a living?"

Dennie wasn't sure she wanted to answer that one.

He swung the chair and was now facing her directly. "Let me tell you."

The Ramberg was not distracting him at all. Somehow she doubted that even one of the Georgia O'Keeffe's would. Or even the real thing. He was a man who could focus well.

"Your dad left the business to David. And all things considered, that was probably a pretty good move on his part. The political life of this city is pretty much an old boys network. Even Lady Jayne Byrne couldn't change that. She could get elected mayor, but she couldn't buck the system. She joined it. So Big Brother David got the business. And that left the three of you out in the cold. Your brother . . . sorry, half brother is a real creep. Treats women like dirt. But I'm sure 'Big Brother' looks out for his little sisters."

"He hardly even recognizes that we exist."

"But he does know how the game is played."

"In spades," she conceded.

"So you three got the rest of the estate. That must have added up to a nice tidy sum."

She said nothing. Her net value was none of his business. The fact was that dad had miscalculated. They each got an apartment and after that there wasn't very much left. Except a partial interest each in D. Cater Construction. But they were each just minority shareholders. And Big Brother owned all the rest. And the only person they could sell to was Brother. And so their million dollar investment meant nothing. Orwell had nothing on this system. David completely controlled the business. Rather than pay dividends, he gave himself a huge salary and bonus and plowed the rest into various ventures. All of which seemed to generate further investments. Ad infinitum. When he died, they'd all be rich. But until then, they were all just middle-class working girls.

"So you all do paralegal work. Free-lance. You're private investigators."

"We're not PIs. We aren't licensed."

"The way I see it, you claim to do legal research. Jessica does the business angle. She's supposed to be a real pro at detecting white-collar crime. What with both an MBA and training as an accountant. She never got licensed as a CPA, though. How come?"

"She never took the test. Dad died. And then she never got around to it."

"She had a nervous breakdown, I understand."

"Two years ago."

"And she's been recuperating ever since. In a private sanatorium."

He knew his facts.

"Where?"

"I don't have to tell you that."

"No, you don't."

"She's my sister. What the heck does her illness have to do with this?" The cardboard frame had worked its way up and was now cutting into her right breast. She tried to shift her weight without being too obvious. If only she'd put on a bra.

"Nothing."

"Outside of Madison. A two-hour drive. I visit her on weekends."

"You don't own a car."

"I borrow a friend's."

"Whose?"

"Am I suspected of something?"

He rotated the chair so that he was looking at the opposite wall, the same one she was looking at. A pair of colorful geometric abstractions filled most of that wall. Paintings she had bought last year.

"Conger," he said.

He really did know Chicago art.

"I like Conger," she informed him. "A lot."

"And Elizabeth? Or should I say Beth? What does she do?"

Little baby sister Beth. Where should she start? "Lit major. The jock of the family. Into weight lifting. No, body building, but works out regularly at the East Bank Club. She does all the footwork. Trails people. Breaks and enters. She even stabbed a guy once. A guy who tried to rape her."

"They were on a date," Ward said.

He obviously knew one heck of a lot more about the three of them than he was telling her. "So what? You think that makes a difference?"

"And it happened in her apartment. She had invited him into her own apartment. What did she think he was going to do there—look at her etchings?"

"Ask her."

"I intend to do just that."

"Those charges were dropped," she reminded him. He had to know all about that.

"Political connections do help."

Dennie was getting tired of the entire conversation. The police were not interested in her; they were interested in her sister.

"Beth was twenty-two then. You would have been twenty-three. She was charged with assault with attempt to do bodily harm."

"I think she wanted to cut off his balls."

"Something like that. But she's not here for me to ask. Or is she?"

"You can check for yourself."

"Thank you . . . ah . . . how do I get in? Do you have a key?"

"There's a door in the kitchen."

"Is it locked?"

"There is no lock."

"Do you mind if I look around?"

"No, I don't, but it's not my apartment." The legal implications of what she had said were not lost on either of them.

Lieutenant Ward walked down the hall and disappeared into the kitchen. Dennie waited about ten seconds then got up, went over to her desk, reached under her sweat shirt, pulled out the cardboard-encased photograph that had been digging into her, gently rubbed her right breast where the cardboard had been jabbing into her, and slipped the picture into one of the bookshelves behind her desk in among a stack of old travelogues. She then sat down at her desk and waited, wondering where the hell Beth was and whether she'd overlooked anything in her apartment. Was there only one picture of Mike, or had there been two?

Tom Ward did not take very long. "She's not there," he said.

That was not exactly a news flash.

"Her bed hasn't been slept in."

Nor was that.

"For days."

Nor that.

"If not longer. And who's Mike?"

"Mike?" Had there been another picture? Damn!

"Yes, Mike."

"Why?"

"There was a message next to her phone. In the living room. It said call Mike at 959-6719. So who is Mike?"

"Why not call and find out?"

"I might just do that."

"Mike's a friend of Beth's." Mike was so much more than a mere friend.

"A good friend?"

"A very good friend." And had been for three years now. Off and on. Mostly on. More stability than Beth had ever known. But none of that was any of this guy's business.

"The kind of friend she might spend the night with?"

Didn't he know he wasn't supposed to end a sentence with a preposition? Even if it was a question. So much for a Chicago public school education.

"Yes," she conceded.

"You wouldn't happen to know Mike's last name?"

"No," she lied. She knew Mike's last name. And Mike's home address. And phone numbers. At work and at home. And neither of them was the number that Tom Ward had found. That was a number Mike had left months ago when they had come back together again. It was the number of some restaurant where they were supposed to meet.

"That's not Mike's number," he said.

"It isn't?"

"Not unless Mike owns Hideo's Sushi Bar."

"I don't think so."

"Neither do I. Do you mind if I look around here?"

"Yes. I mind."

"I could get a search warrant."

"Maybe you could; maybe you couldn't. I'm not a suspect, am I?"

Ward got up to leave. The phone rang. Dennie grabbed the receiver. "Yes?" she said hurriedly.

"Ms. Cater," the voice sang out.

"Speaking."

"Laundly leady," the voice continued.

"Thank you."

"Who was that?" he asked.

"My laundry is back."

"When your sister gets back, tell her we're looking for her."

"I'll bet she has already figured that out."

"I'll bet she has, too."

"Good luck in finding your killer."

"If she contacts you, let us know."

"I will," she lied. She knew that Beth had already contacted her. Dennie didn't have any laundry at the dry cleaners. The dry cleaners acted as an unofficial message center and drop-off point for its regular customers. Beth had obviously been there and dropped off something for her. Overnight. Before the laundry opened. That meant she knew she had to lie low.

Why? What exactly had happened to John Doran?

Tom Ward was standing in the hallway now.

"Tom?"

"Yeah?"

"I'm scared. For Beth. She might be in some sort of danger. What happened?"

"She was seen outside Doran's place early yesterday evening. He was inside seeing patients. His last patient was at eight. When he didn't get home, his wife got worried. She called the police around eleven-thirty. The local cop got there at eleven-forty-five. Doran was already dead. He'd been murdered. Stabbed. He was lying naked on the couch in his office with a knife sticking out of his back. He'd been dead for well over an hour."

"How do you know Beth was even in his office?"

"We're guessing. We knew she'd been hanging around watching him, off and on. She'd even had an appointment with him. She was listed in his appointment book."

She had that appointment, not Beth. D. Cater. Not B. Cater or E. Cater.

"And the secretary confirmed seeing her outside yesterday evening when she went home."

"What time was that?"

"About eight."

"So what does that prove?"

"Not much."

"So. What's your case?"

"It was the same kind of knife."

"Same kind of knife?"

"Yeah, just like the one she used before. And I'll bet it has the same fingerprints on it."

"Maybe he tried to. . . ," she stopped. She knew that made no sense.

"Whoever he was making love to killed him." He paused, "You wouldn't happen to have your sister's daily diary, would you? Or her address book?"

"No."

"I didn't think so."

She started to close the door.

"How come you knew that it was John Doran who had been killed?"

"I . . . I got a call."

"Political connections only go so far. Even in this town. Don't count on them to save her neck this time."

"She didn't kill him. She had no reason to."

"I no longer believe that people have to have reasons for what they do. That's for whodunits. Motive. Christ. Most murderers don't have real motives. Not ones that would stand up in a good mystery story."

He turned to leave. She once again felt the chill. As usual, it was not just the cold air from the hallway that was invading her apartment. Suddenly he turned around once again. "Your dad's influence only goes so far."

"I know, damn it."

"There are always limits. To anyone's influence."

She converted a shudder into a shrug. It was easier than saying anything.

"How was she killed?"

"Who?"

"Your father's first wife?"

"I don't know. Some kind of accident."

"What kind?" he persisted.

"I don't know. I never did. I wasn't there. Hell, I wasn't even born yet. I couldn't have been. He was still married to her. If she hadn't had that accident, I would never have been born. Nor my sisters. What difference does it make?"

"That kind of difference."

"You are a suspicious. . . ." Her voiced drifted off. It had made a difference.

"How long afterwards?"

"A few months," softly.

"Hm."

"What's that supposed to mean?"

"Nothing. But he was not exactly the long-grieving widower. In my business it's always the husband."

"All of life is not your business," she cursed at him, clenching her fists to keep from doing something more violent with them. Dad. Her dad. How could this SOB say what he was saying? "My father wouldn't have hurt a flea. Ever."

"We weren't discussing fleas."

"Go away."

And he did.

Chapter
III

She had to think of something else. Anything else. But what? Jessie. Beth. The three sisters. The three weird sisters. her two sisters. Two. *Racemic.* That was the word. *Racemers.* Their two apartments were *racemers* of one another. Probably from the Latin. Symmetric. Like the leaves of a fern. Mirror images.

Dennie watched as Lieutenant Tom Ward stood waiting in the hallway opposite the elevators. In time, an elevator arrived and its door opened. The policeman got in, turned around, and disappeared behind the closing doors. Without so much as a wave. He was wrong. It had been an accident. Accidents happened. Even in her family. Even if it hadn't been, he was still wrong. It wasn't always the fathers who were to blame.

Racemers. Beth would be so proud of her for remembering such an obscure word. And even its derivation. She closed the door, cutting off the source of the frigid air that had been enveloping her. She felt no warmer. No better. No more at ease. No safer. Safer.

Beth! Where was she? How was she? Was she safe? Was she okay? If only she had heard from her. Then Dennie remembered. "Laundly leady."

She dashed back into her bedroom, pulling off her sweat shirt as she went along. Her right breast still ached. She pulled on her bra and snapped it behind her. Then she yanked off the sweat pants and pulled on some panties. What to wear? A business suit. What else? Dad had liked her in business suits. If only the chill would leave her marrow. She reached into the closet and pulled out a blouse and a suit. In no time she was dressed and brushing her teeth. Then her hair.

The phone rang.

"Three Sisters," she said. Very business-like. Almost cool. God, she hated that word.

"Do you do wiretaps?" the voice asked. It sounded like Sean's voice.

"No."

"Some people do." It was Sean. And he had not been asking an idle question.

"We don't."

"Do you find missing people."

"Sometimes."

"Successfully?"

"I think so."

"Good."

There was a pause. Was the tap already on her line? Probably. If not yet, it would be soon. Having connections sure helped in this city. It probably helped in any city. Only more so in Chicago. Where clout had been perfected. If not invented.

"Do you know anything about search warrants?" Sean asked her.

"Yes."

"What does *contiguous* mean?"

What was this, an English lesson? "Adjoining," she replied.

"Not separated," he said. "Like no locks."

Like their kitchen doorway. It had no lock. Two for one. Two apartments on a single search warrant. So that was what *contiguous* meant. "Do you know what *racemic* means?" she asked.

"Hell, no."

"I do," she said, and started to hang up.

"Call if you get some work," he said.

Nice and ambiguous. Except it was not ambiguous at all. She should call from a line that wasn't tapped. She would. When she got some news. That is if she got any news.

She heard a click and hung up. Good ol' Sean. Thank God he still loved Jessica and, because of that love, cared for the rest of them. Not loved her in a passionate way. Not now. But like best friends. Old roommates. Which is what they were. A nice, ambiguous euphemism, that. Jessie and Sean had been roommates one summer. She had never seen them together. She was in Chicago that summer, but she spent those months by herself, trying to figure out what she wanted to do with her life. She had finished college. She had to do something. During the days she wandered around the art galleries and museums and bookstores. In the evenings she read the books she had bought, isolated from everyone. Even from her sisters. Trying to become herself. One and independent. She was not just one of a set of triplets. She was an individual. So she learned about herself. And about Chicago's homegrown art. At first she didn't particularly like either. Then mom died. And dad got sick. And in the Fall, he got sicker. Then he died. That seemed like a lifetime ago. Three lifetimes ago. If not longer. There had been so many changes in their lives. In Jessie's? Did she still love Sean? Was he a father figure to her? When she and Sean. . . ? That was crazy. Insane. And getting her nowhere. Slowly. Like a Chekhov play.

She had to get rid of the appointment book, the daily diary. And Beth's address book. But she might also need them.

Where? Not inside her contiguous apartment. She had learned that much from Sean's little vocabulary lesson.

What would Beth do? She was a lot better at this. No wonder Mike loved her so. Mike was sure as hell no father figure. She missed dad so. And that was normal. They all did. Except Beth sometimes. When she was in one of her angry spells. Why did she get so damn angry? Poor Beth. All Dennie had to do was to think like Beth. That was harder than it seemed. Two sisters were rarely so different. Beth! What would she do? When they had been the three Cater triplets it had been easy to think like Beth. And like Jessie. Was it their age? How different were the minds of adolescent girls? Not as different as those of three adult women in their late twenties. Especially when each of them treasured and needed those differences. And the separation they represented. And the independence. In a way Ward had made the right reference. The Three Weird Sisters. Out of Shakespeare, not Chekhov. And now one of them was in trouble. And Dennie was the only one who could help her.

What would Beth do? Where would she. . . ? Bingo. Dennie knew. The solution was obvious. Thanks to Beth. Dennie went back into her walk-in closet and packed her dirty clothes into a large cloth laundry bag. She then took two smaller laundry bags down from the shelf. She crossed back into her bedroom and opened the middle drawer of her dresser. She took a stack of clean folded clothes from her dresser. Some sweat shirts, a couple of cotton T-shirts, and a pair of shorts. She folded them neatly into the two clean laundry bags. Not too much. A light load into each.

Back to the living room. To her desk. To the appointment book. She put it into one of the partially filled laundry bags. She opened the address book and checked Mike's phone number.

O'Rourke, M. The entry seemed so formal. She'd remembered the numbers correctly. She put the address book into the same laundry bag and then folded both partially filled bags into her big laundry bag. She was ready to go.

✳✳✳✳

The dry cleaners was on the first floor shopping mall that stretched the length of their building. She walked down the wood-lined staircase and entered the small mall. The hallway was deserted. The cleaners was opposite the video store. There were already several customers in the video store. At eight thirty on a Saturday morning. Why not? Luckily there was no one inside the dry cleaners.

She pushed the door open and went into the cleaners.

"Miss Cater," the little Oriental girl said. The dry cleaners was a family affair. And on Saturday morning, the daughter ran the counter while the father sat at the sewing machine in back and watched over her and the customers. It was the only day of the week that the mother wasn't also there. The little girl must have been all of eleven years old at the very most. And a very little, very bright eleven. With coal black eyes and hair and a golden complexion. She ran the cash register perfectly and figured change faster than it did. And smart enough to call all three of them "Miss Cater." That way she never made a mistake. All Caucasian women probably looked the same to her. Especially tall, lanky blondes who were about the same height, the same weight, and the same age.

"Hi, Linn," Dennie said. It had been the father who had called and left the message. He sat in the back, a silent visage.

"There is no laundry, Miss Cater," she said, in perfect English.

"I think there's a package for me," Dennie said, lifting her laundry onto the counter and pulling out the two smaller bags. Her back and the large bag on the counter would completely block the view of anyone in the corridor outside the cleaners. And certainly of anyone in that video outlet. She had to lean over the bag to see the little girl.

The girl handed her a small paper bag. "Dennie Cater, 2B," was written on it in Beth's left-handed scrawl.

Dennie took the paper bag from her. There was a videotape inside. She stuffed the bag into one of the two small laundry bags. The one that had only clean clothes. The other small bag she gave to the little girl. "This is for my sister," she said. "Hold it for her."

"Which one is she?" the girl asked innocently.

"Beth," she said, "2A."

Linn took out a receipt and wrote "Beth Cater, 2A" on it and pinned it to the laundry.

"And the laundry is mine."

The little girl took another receipt and wrote "Denise Cater, 2B" on it and heaved the big bag off the counter.

Dennie turned and walked out just like any other customer, carrying a bag of clean clothes. Pretty good for a rank amateur. No private eye could have done it more smoothly. Then why did she feel like she was acting in some third-rate satire that was about to flop? And none too soon. And why was her heart pounding?

Not like any other customer. She hadn't paid. "I'll pay you when I pick up the next load," she called out.

The little girl didn't know what to say.

"I call when laundly leady," the father called out to her.

The mall was still empty. Had anyone seen her? Watched her? Did anyone care? Someone did. And that someone was a killer. A murderer. Who? She hadn't an inkling.

✳✳✳✳

The image on her TV screen was that of a man's backside. The man was completely naked. The camera seemed to be focused on the lower part of his spine. It was centered about four inches above the top end of the crease of his buttocks. And about six inches below the handle of a knife. It was a wooden handle of a butcher knife and the knife was sticking out of his back. Out of the left side of his back, just to the left of his spine and just above his rib cage. It had definitely entered his chest. And done some harm. Red blood had collected at the base of the knife. Not much blood.

The man was not moving.

Nor was the camera.

And there was no noise. That had to be the volume. She turned up the volume on the TV until the machine hummed, but there still was no sound so she turned it back down until the hum disappeared. She repeated the same process with the remote for the VCR. Still no sound.

The body still hadn't moved. Nor had the knife, nor the blood. As far as she could tell that meant that he was no longer bleeding. To go along with the fact that he was no longer breathing. Two facts that fit together quite well. Neither of which was a good sign for this naked man.

Even his feet were bare, she noted.

He was obviously dead. Killed by that knife in his chest.

She concentrated on the butcher knife that was sticking out of the wound that was no longer bleeding. It was angled to the right at about sixty degrees. The murderer had come to him from his right side. No. That obviously had not been what had happened. He . . . and she assumed that he was John Doran. An obvious conclusion. It didn't require the logical powers of a Sherlock Holmes. How many men could have been killed by butcher knives in the last few days? Not that many. At least not in full view of an overhead camera. It had to be the body of the reluctant therapist. Now the naked therapist. Naked and dead. He wouldn't have to testify now. He was off the hook. Bad pun. She tried to reconstruct what must have happened. Doran had probably not been sleeping in his office like that and been stabbed from behind by an unknown intruder. No one would buy a story like that. Besides it was physically impossible. The couch was against a wall. A solid wall.

But the angle. What did it mean? That the murderer had been below him. The murder blow had been an arc. The arc started from below this naked man. While they were. . . . Conan Doyle had never described such a crime.

The murderer had to have reached behind him and stabbed him on his left side. An arc-like movement. That explained the angle.

There wasn't much blood around the wound. The butcher knife must have gone directly into his left lung. As far as she could tell there was no evidence of a struggle. All she could see was a single wound. No scratches. Nothing else.

The knife blade must have gone into more than just his lung. It must have gone directly into his heart. With all but surgical accuracy. And a good deal of force.

And instantaneous death.

More or less. That Conan Doyle would have understood. He was a physician.

Dennie made a fist and pretended she was holding that butcher knife in her right hand. And she swung it around in a violent stabbing movement. A semi-circular arc coming to rest on her own left breast. At a sixty degree angle. Into her heart. From the front. No, the anatomic term was not *front*. It was *anterior.* From the anterior approach.

Was the angle correct?

That depended on their position.

Missionary, she assumed. And how thick was he? Two ten, two twenty. Overweight but not that obese. She'd reached around men that thick. Not often. And certainly not recently.

Sixty degrees was about right.

No. It was all wrong. She was totally wrong. She was sixty degrees off. Dennie let her right hand fall back down and her fist fall open. She held her hands out in front of her, both hands open, her palms facing up. She then shifted the imaginary knife to her left hand with a simple toss. She caught it in her left hand, her fist closing down on the handle. The arc had come to rest just inside her right breast, which was still tender.

They had been racemers. A racemic mixture. Left leg over right leg. Left chest over right chest. Left shoulder on right shoulder. And left arm into left back from the left side, at a sixty degree angle.

The murderer had been left-handed.

Not murderer. It had not been a murderer. It had been a murderess.

If it had been a man. . . . It couldn't have been a man, naked and below him. It had to have been a woman. A naked woman. Or at least with her skirt up to her waist. A left-handed murderess.

A left-handed woman. A woman who had killed him while. . . . Coitus interruptus maximus. Who said she didn't know any Latin?

Beth was left-handed. And she had stabbed one man. With a butcher knife. One very much like this one she was staring at. Weren't all butcher knives pretty much the same?

"Hi." The single word startled Dennie. It was Beth's voice, coming out of the TV set. She sounded winded, as if she were catching her breath. "I'm back. I was just putting fresh tape in Doran's set-up. In case you didn't recognize him. That's Doran. John Doran. Not exactly his best side. Just his most appropriate. His camera is fixed in the ceiling just like you thought. Right behind that little window. The actual recording goes on in a little alcove behind his desk. It's a very professional set-up. A fixed remote camera."

Despite the addition of a sound track, the scene never changed. The camera might well be fixed, but it was hard to call it remote.

"The camera never moves. It just focuses on his couch," the voice said coldly.

She was so good at analysis. And at observation.

"He was dead when I got here. I didn't kill him. But it sure looks like he was killed by a left-handed woman while they were making love. Now I ask you, would I let a fat slob like that make love to me?"

It was, Dennie assumed, a rhetorical question. Dennie knew the answer. Beth wouldn't. She might. She had. But not Beth. She was a fitness freak.

"Mike would kill me."

True. Mike might. Cops could get violent when enraged. And when jealous. Mike was certainly the jealous type. That was one of the reasons their relationship had had so many ups and downs.

"He was dead when I got here," she repeated, "with that knife sticking out of him and the little pool of dark red blood. I got in through the front door. I sort of borrowed his receptionist's keys. Not sort of. I did. To use the bathroom. And when I gave them back, she was a couple keys short."

So she, too, had been to see Doran. Why? They had agreed that Dennie would see him as a potential patient and that Beth would play detective. At least that was what Dennie had thought they had agreed to. That had been their overall plan.

"She never uses her door keys. Doran gets here at nine and she comes in around eleven. She leaves at six. He sees patients . . . sorry, clients. If you can call them all clients. He sees them until eight or nine. Maybe later. She leaves around six. She still probably doesn't know I have her keys, which I don't. They are in the bag, taped to the bottom. There are two of them."

Dennie reached for the paper bag and felt inside it. The keys were there. Two of them.

"Put them on your key ring. A search warrant for my apartment will include your apartment but not your person."

Beth was sure way ahead of her on this.

"It looks like he was making love to a woman. A left-handed woman who stabbed him. In media res, so to speak. And I do mean media. And I am left-handed! And it is a butcher knife."

"Fifteen percent of all women are left-handers."

Dennie knew that.

"And we don't know he was making love."

True, there was no proof of that. Or at least none that Dennie could see. There might be another reason for his nakedness. She always slept naked. Even when she slept alone. Which was almost always. No, it was always.

But on the couch of his office? What other reason could there be?

"Or if he was making it, that it was to a woman."

Not a woman? That was not an alternative that had occurred to Dennie.

"It could have been a left-handed man."

How?

"Use your imagination."

Dennie tried.

"Or a right-hander."

A right-hander?

"Of either sex."

Of either sex? How the hell?

"Think about it. Recreate the scene. Remember things you've done. Movies you've seen. Books you've read. Your fantasies. Even you ought to be able to. . . ."

She was. She could. Beth was right. Once you'd assumed that the obvious need not be true then the possibilities were enormous. They included everyone else in the world big enough and strong enough to wield a butcher knife.

"I'll be okay. I won't be home for a while. So I'd appreciate it if you could call Mike for me."

She could do that. Once she got to a phone without a tap on it. She was already planning to do it.

"At home. Tell Mike not to worry. Mike is such a worrywart. More like a little old lady than a cop."

Easily done.

"And don't worry."

Not so easily done.

"I'll be in touch. Hasta la vesta."

Her Spanish was as terrible as it had been in high school. But Dennie knew what she meant.

The voice stopped. John Doran's body continued to fill her TV screen. It was still not moving. Or breathing. Or bleeding. And it was still pierced by a butcher knife surrounded by a small pool of violet blood.

Dennie pressed FAST FORWARD. The tracking streak cut his body in half, obliterating the butcher knife and then the entire screen was filled by a light pattern of snow.

Virgin tape.

The show was over. Dennie pushed STOP. The tape stopped. She pushed EJECT. The tape came out of the machine. Dennie took it and went over to her desk. She found a label, pasted it on the tape, and wrote "Three Sisters Vacation." Where? "Spain," and put it on a book shelf filled with other tapes. Between "Three Sisters—Italy" and "Three Sisters—Portugal." Geographic. Not alphabetic.

Poor Beth. On the run. Isolated. Alone. She had to be frightened again. A frightened little girl in a grownup body. With no one to turn to. No. That wasn't true. Beth had her. And Mike. Mike. Dennie had to call Mike. All Beth had was her and Mike. But who did Dennie have? Tears collected in both of her eyes. Damn it! She didn't have time to feel sorry for herself. That never helped. She had things to do. And miles to go before she. . . .

Dennie crossed the street and walked toward a small storefront coffee shop. This was where Beth usually had breakfast since even making coffee was too much like cooking. And she had no toaster.

It was warm for February. High forties. No wind at all. Why had it seemed so cold before? The street was almost empty. She'd forgotten it was Saturday. And it was still early for most Chicagoans. Just barely nine.

The lady behind the counter smiled at her. "How's your sister?" she asked.

"Fine. Toast me a pecan roll, please. And coffee. Where's your phone?"

"In back, across from the washrooms."

Dennie nodded.

"You make your calls, honey, and I'll bring your roll and coffee to a table."

"Thanks."

First she called Mike. After four rings a harsh, gravelly voice began to talk. It wasn't Mike's. It was some sports announcer. Harry Carey? Or someone impersonating him? He was the voice of the Chicago Cubs. He used to be the voice of the Chicago White Sox, or was it the other way around? And did that matter? It undoubtedly did, to some people. Was that really Harry? It was hard to be certain. Mike was a crazy Cub fan. She'd forgotten that.

"Here comes the pitch. Santo swings. It's a line drive over the second baseman's head. Into right field."

My God. An entire play by play.

"Williams rounds second. He's heading for third. Clemente has the ball. Williams is half way to third. Clemente's throw is on the way to third. Williams slides.

"And he's out. Billy Williams is out. And so is Mike. Leave a message when you hear the next crack of a bat."

Crack.

Beep.

"This is Dennie, Mike. Beth is fine. She wanted me to call you. She sends her love." She hadn't. That was hard for her to do. Even to Mike. Why? She loved Mike. Then why? If Dennie only knew the answer to that one.

The second call was to Sean Keneally. At his office.

"Where you calling from?"

"A pay phone," she reassured him. "I heard from Elizabeth," she began, remembering his preference for real names. No nicknames for him. "She told me that she didn't kill him."

"Not exactly an unbiased source of information."

"Stop sounding like a lawyer," Dennie admonished him.

"I am a lawyer."

"That's no excuse. Elizabeth is innocent."

"I wouldn't go that far," Sean contradicted her.

"Of this crime."

He said nothing.

"Doran was dead when she got there."

"But she was there? At Doran's?"

"Yes."

"And I suppose the police can place her there?"

"Probably."

"And he was stabbed," Sean continued.

"Yes."

"With a knife," he persisted.

"Yes, a butcher knife," she concurred.

"The same kind of butcher knife?"

"I guess so," she admitted. How many kinds are there?

"No guessing allowed."

"Yes," she admitted.

"In media res, so to speak."

"So to speak." But who the hell spoke that way? No one she knew.

"By a left-handed woman whom he was. . . ."

"We don't know he was doing that."

"Don't we?"

"Or that even if he was making it, that he was making it with a woman."

"Not with a woman? What the hell are you talking about? How the. . . ."

"It could have been a left-handed man," she interrupted him.

"How?" he reiterated.

"Use your imagination."

"I'm trying."

"Or a right-hander!"

"A right-hander?"

"Of either sex."

"How the hell?"

"Think about it. Recreate the scene. Remember things you've done. Movies you've seen, books you've read. Your fantasies. Even you ought to be able to. . . ." She stopped. He had made love to Jessie. Jessie had never been exactly a blushing virgin. At least not that late in her life.

"You may be right," he conceded. "Once you assume that the obvious might not be true, then the various possibilities are staggering."

"A whole Kama Sutra of variations," she suggested.

"And then some." He seemed to be relishing the various options.

"So how do we prove that Beth didn't do it?" she asked.

"All we have to do is raise a reasonable benefit of doubt. Beyond a reasonable doubt."

"More lawyer talk," she said sarcastically.

He knew she was right. According to Sean's sources, Ward was pretty convinced that Elizabeth Cater had murdered John Doran.

"You can't expect cops to go beyond the obvious. Much less beyond the Kama Sutra." Mike excluded, she hoped.

"Don't underestimate Tom Ward," Sean warned her. "He's supposed to be very good. And very thorough. So be careful. He's decided to let the arrest warrant drop for now."

"Why?"

"Your family still has a lot of clout in this town. But that doesn't mean that he won't go after her. He's just not going to arrest her. For the time being."

Chalk up one more for dear ol' dad. Clout from beyond the grave. What had Anthony said about what had been buried with Caesar? What the hell did Anthony know?

"What are we going to do to help Beth?" she wondered aloud.

"You'll just have to prove that somebody else did it."

"Who?"

"Leslie's stepfather is a hell of a good suspect, for starters. He knew that Doran was her therapist. That's how the whole lawsuit started. She went to see Doran. He dredged up what the old man had done to her. And he thinks that Doran was going to testify against him at trial."

The son of a bitch! Raped his own daughter. No, stepdaughter. He ought to be drawn and quartered. No. Something even more cruel and unusual than that. For those rapes. To say nothing of mere murder. She had to control herself.

"Why would he think that Doran was going to testify?"

"I listed Doran as a witness."

"But he wasn't going to testify."

"You and I know that. So did Leslie. But her stepfather didn't."

"So kill Doran and the case might go away."

"It's a motive."

What had Ward said? Motives were for paperback thrillers. If they could prove that he was guilty, the State would punish him for murder. Not the rack, but life in prison wasn't a picnic. Someone ought to cut off his balls and stuff them down his throat.

"And he's not the only one," Sean continued. "Take her mom."

"Her mom? Was she going to be a witness too?"

"A defendant. Leslie had just amended her complaint. Her mom had been an accomplice. She had held her. Forced her. Helped him. She even participated."

"What!"

"Leslie had another session with Doran yesterday. After she left here, she remembered more. And. . . ." He paused. "Let's just say Leslie amended the complaint."

"Did her mom know that?"

"We served the papers on her late yesterday afternoon."

Motive. Leslie's mom had a motive too. Dennie was beginning to think like a detective in a whodunit. Was that good or bad? It probably depended. "That makes two, I guess," she said.

"Don't sound so convinced. There are undoubtedly others."

"Accomplices."

"No, suspects. It may not be a coincidence that Doran was killed when somebody started investigating his life."

"What do you mean?"

"Elizabeth was looking for dirt on Doran. And his dirt may have been someone else's mud."

"Whose?"

"That, my dear Denise, is your problem. Yours and Tom Ward's. Good luck."

Her coffee was waiting for her on a table in the corner. So was the pecan roll. The coffee was still warm. The pecan roll wasn't. She pulled off a strip and dunked it into her coffee. The butter formed a thin yellowish ring on the coffee. Denise absently took a bite of the pecan roll.

Someone else's mud. Whose? Only John Doran knew whose. And he was dead. And maybe that was the reason. A dead man told no tales. But his tapes sure as hell might, and she had a key to his office and all of those videotapes. Some of which might not be so remote after all.

She dunked again and took another bite. This one tasted better. Had Tom Ward looked beyond the obvious? The Kama Sutra? Had he read it? Would he like to? Would he like a personal introduction?

It had been far too long.

Chapter
IV

It would take her only a few moments to negotiate her car rental and there would be no paperwork. Something else she'd learned from Beth. Neither of them owned cars. Cabs were cheap. And easy to put on their expense accounts. And parking was such a hassle. And it was easier to let their dates do the driving. That made them feel more masculine. Did Tom Ward like to drive? Or was a day in a squad car enough for him? She walked back to her building from the coffee shop, but instead of going up the one flight of stairs to her apartment, she went through a small doorway on the side of the lobby and down one flight into what had once been the basement delivery docks of the old printshop. The half underground level now served as the building's indoor parking garage, complete with one gas pump and a service area for washing cars, changing tires, or carrying out other minor repairs. She strode past the service area and opened the door to the small office.

A.C. was on duty. It seemed as if he were always there. He was officially in charge of the garage. He was also in charge of the unofficial rental service. A.C. was at his desk looking at a copy of some car magazine. At least it wasn't *Hustler.*

"Ma'am. Whichever of the ma'ams you is. How can we help you?"

"I need a car, A.C."

"I got a whole garage full. What kind you needs?"

"Cut the act," she said.

"Okay, Dennie. How's Beth? I haven't seen her in weeks. She staying out of trouble?"

"I sure hope so."

He reached into his pocket and pulled out a set of car keys and handed them to her. She in turn handed him a twenty.

He shook his head so she pulled out another twenty. A.C. smiled.

That was more than a cost of living increase. "What kind of car am I driving this week?" she asked him. "It ought to be pretty special to justify forty bucks a day."

"An old 'vette. I just put a new motor in it. You'll love it." A.C. made most of his money rebuilding junks and then selling them. That was what he had told Beth, at least.

What, she wondered, was a vet? A car that had been through the war? Through Desert Storm? Some real . . . beater? That was the word. A rehabed beater.

He smiled at her dilemma. "It's the red car behind you. I just finished tuning it." He pointed to a low-slung red sports car that was in the shop area. The kind of car that you fell into.

"That's a vet?" she asked.

"As in Corvette," A.C. smiled at her.

They walked over to the 'vette. She half climbed and half fell into it. She felt as if she were sitting on a couch that was far too low for sitting. Her skirt had pulled up far above her knees. After nodding his approval of her thighs, A.C. gave her a few instructions, a couple of warnings, and then asked, "Beth still heavy with that cop?"

"How did you. . .?"

"They drove in here a couple of times."

Who else knew?

"Mike? Right?" A.C. continued.

She nodded.

"They do make a nice-looking couple."

"So did Bonnie and Clyde," she quipped.

He laughed.

Why had she said that?

✳✳✳✳

The fastest route to Glencoe would have been to take the expressways. The Eisenhower to the Kennedy to the Edens. Whoever he had been. Speed was not the issue today. No one was expecting her. And she wasn't certain they'd welcome her if they were. She needed some time to clear her head. And what better way than a nice quiet drive? So Dennie took Lake Shore Drive. She loved driving along the lakefront. Even in February. The lake was a light blue-gray. The waves crashed heavily against the rocks. The water looked cold and choppy. Foreboding. Hostile. Aggressive. But not in a threatening way. More like a friendly guard dog. One that would never bite a friend. The lake was her old friend. There were no boats out on it. And no one was on the tan beaches. And there was no activity in the blue-green lagoons. It was Chicago on a bleak Saturday in the middle of winter. She felt better just by watching it all.

And the 'vette handled beautifully. She was beginning to understand why men felt the way they did about sports cars. It was so damn responsive. Was that what the male fantasy was all about? If you couldn't find a responsive woman, find a responsive car. But the shrinks said that sports cars were phallic symbols. Part of some sort of penis envy. That had never made much sense to Dennie. Did A.C.'s car magazine have a centerfold? With its hood wide open? Or its trunk? Or was that just too kinky?

Kinky. That was the word Leslie had used. To describe Doran's videos. Kinky. And Leslie knew about kinky. From bitter experience. Had John Doran been kinky? Had his kinkiness gone sour? Had it turned into murder? Dennie gazed down at the panel. She was going seventy-five. It didn't feel like a mile over forty. She slowed down to fifty. The road was marked fifty-five. And she was in no particular hurry.

At Bryn Mawr, Lake Shore Drive left the shore of Lake Michigan and turned landward to become Sheridan Road. Named after General Phil Sheridan. Of Civil War fame. Really after Fort Sheridan. An army base, north of Chicago. And this was the old road north from Chicago to Fort Sheridan. A modified frontier trail that wound its way through the northern end of Chicago and then into the suburbs. But not along the lakefront. At least not for most of its itinerary. The riparian right no longer belonged to the driver.

Into Evanston. Past Northwestern University. She never drove past the campus without pangs of regret that she had not gone to college there and stayed nearer home. Even on a cold gray day, the campus looked inviting. Warm. Friendly. And far less threatening than the neighborhood around Columbia had been. Just a few blocks from Harlem.

She had, she realized, never met a murderer before. Or a murderess. Not that she was certain that that was what she was about to do. She was on her way to drop in on Leslie's mother and stepfather and the Krollers were the only two suspects so far with motives that made any sense to her. Sean had said that there would probably be other suspects. One of them had to be more than a mere suspect. But who? She had her candidate. Kroller. Child-molesting bastard. Just thinking about him made her sick to her stomach.

❋❋❋❋

Once Sheridan Road twisted its way into Glencoe, Dennie took a glance at the handy pocket map she always kept in her purse. Thank God her Dad had taught her how to read road maps. One quick glance and a couple of U-turns and she negotiated her way to Leslie's house. Except it wasn't Leslie's house. It was Leslie's parents' house.

The house was on the lakefront, set well back from the street. It had a long, circular driveway, all but hidden by trees that finally led to the house itself. A house that just didn't fit there. The long columns in front were more out of Virginia than Illinois. Monticello, not Chicago. Mount Vernon, not Glencoe.

Those weren't the right models. Not the Revolutionary War. The Civil War. The antebellum South. Not Mount Vernon at all. Tara. In all its glory. But a Tara in the wrong place. To say nothing of the wrong era. The house had probably been built right before World War II, when *Gone with the Wind* was the rage. It was big. Probably as big as Tara. Behind it was the lake. Quieter now. Less foreboding. Less choppy. Bluer. But no more friendly.

Dennie went up to the ten foot high front door. It was white, of course. What else? She pushed the bell. It was not just a simple bell. Chimes, of course. Pealing. She half expected the original sound track. With full orchestra. And chorus.

The door came open. A mammy, she was willing to bet. She would have lost that bet. She was a he. And he looked more like a bodyguard. Male. Late twenties. Six four. Two fifty. Built like the proverbial linebacker. Black. Clean-shaven head. He'd stand out in any crowd. Even a crowd of linebackers.

"Can I help you?" he asked.

"Are the Krollers in?" she asked after identifying herself. When Leslie's mom married William Kroller, her mom became a Kroller. Leslie never did. Her dad had been alive and living, somewhere in California. He was still alive as far as Dennie knew. He sent Leslie a present on her birthday every year. That was it. Some father. At least he never. . . .

"Are they expecting you?" the linebacker asked.

"No," she admitted.

The dark eyes were scrutinizing her from head to toe. Her and her car. "I love 'vettes," he said. "Especially classic Stingrays like that one. They are so responsive. Like a beautiful woman ought to be. Someday I'm going to get me one."

Dennie realized that his statement was not ambiguous. It was not a beautiful woman he wanted to get.

"Who rebuilt the engine?" he asked.

"A.C.," she said.

He nodded. "Figures. He rebuilt a motor for a friend of mine. My name's Eller. Horace Eller. I'll see if they are receiving. Ms. . . . ."

"Cater. Denise Cater," she repeated, pulling a card out of her pocket.

"Three Sisters Limited," he read aloud. He looked at the car again. "They'll be in. Any friend of A.C.'s couldn't be all bad. Come on into the living room. I'll announce you," he said, stepping back to allow her in and then closing the door behind her.

He didn't offer to take her coat. Times had changed. It wasn't Reconstruction any more. And this wasn't Georgia.

The living room was not designed for living. It was huge. Probably thirty by thirty-five. At least a thousand square feet. The ceiling had to be thirty feet high. And right in the middle of the ceiling there was a large, gaudy, cut-glass chandelier hanging down and occupying much of the first eight to ten feet. The chandelier gave new meaning to the phrase "a ceiling made of glass." Entirely new. And much more costly. The furniture looked as if it had once been part of a set for *Gone with the Wind.* Rich. Red. Opulent. Overstuffed. And yet cold and austere. Antebellum Atlanta. Formal. Lush. Pretentious. More pretentious than tasteful. Early Victorian opulence. Antebellum rococo, if there was such a phrase. Either Tara or a New Orleans bordello. And covered with plastic. Look, but don't ever touch.

Could someone make a dress out of the drapes?

"The interior decorator did the sets for *Gone with the Wind,*" a woman said.

Dennie turned, startled. She hadn't heard anyone enter the room.

"That chandelier was in the movie," she continued coldly. "Everyone asks."

The woman appeared to be in her late forties. Maybe early fifties. She was not tall, but she sure as hell had a presence. Jet black hair, cut full, about shoulder length and flecked with just enough gray to let you know that this was a woman who didn't need to hide anything, who was in complete control. Of a lot more than just her own life.

Mrs. Kroller slipped on a pair of half-glasses that she'd been holding and looked at the card. "Ms. Cater," she said, "to what do I owe the pleasure of this visit?"

"I'm a friend of Leslie's."

"That is not exactly a declaration of undying loyalty."

Time for another tactic. "I'm also looking into the death of John Doran."

"Good riddance."

Mrs. Kroller continued to look at the card. As if it should remind her of something. "From the Andrews Sisters, I suppose."

"Yes," she lied. "My mother wanted to name us Patty, Maxine, and Laverne. My father wouldn't let her."

"Good for him," a voice bellowed out, catching her completely by surprise. "They were three of the ugliest broads."

"William, please."

"My wife thinks *broads* is a dirty word," he said. "I'm William Kroller. I live here too." He crossed the room, extended his hand to her. Dennie's hand shot out automatically. She tried to pull it back. Before she could he grabbed it and shook it vigorously. "Who are you?" he asked.

She had touched him. He had touched her. Nausea built up in the back of her throat. She wanted to vomit. To rid herself. . . . Control. She had to stay in control of herself. It had been a mere handshake. That was all. "Dennie Cater. I'm here because. . . ."

"I know why you're here."

She was certain that they did.

"You belong to Donald Cater. Right?"

Donald. Not David. Father. Not son. "Yes."

"I thought so. I met your dad a couple of times. Some damn dinner we both had to go to. Some sort of artsy-fartsy affair. In monkey suits. I liked your Dad. Even if he pretended to like that kind of dinner. We even did a little business. Not much. By the way, your brother's a creep. In case you didn't already know."

Anyone who thought that couldn't be all bad.

"But who am I to criticize anybody? I rape little girls."

Dennie could think of nothing to say in response. That was the charge in Leslie's suit. A charge they had been retained to help prove. A charge she knew had to be true.

He plopped himself down in the one chair that looked as if it had been used more than once. "You mind if I smoke a cigar? I know my wife does, so I won't ask her."

She did. "No," she said. Why not foster a little discord? Wasn't that a detective's job? Stir things up and see what came to the surface.

He pulled a cigar out of the pocket of his double knit pullover, stuck it in his mouth and bit down on it but did not light it. "The joke's on me. My doctors say I can't smoke. No good for my ticker. All I can do is chew on 'em. And suck on 'em a bit. All too damn Freudian for me. A cigar is just a cigar."

He pulled the cigar out of his mouth, looked at it, rolled it in his fingers, very sensually, and then put it back in his mouth, almost nostalgically. "Sit down," he said.

She did. On one of the overstuffed, underutilized opulent couches. When was the formal dress ball going to start? And why hadn't she remembered to wear a gown?

Mrs. Kroller had not budged. She was still holding Dennie's business card but she had taken off her glasses.

"So what can I tell you?" he asked. "I didn't kill the SOB. I didn't have him killed. I could have, I suppose. I know people. In my business, who doesn't? Some of the same people your dad knew."

"What business is that?" she asked, trying to change the direction of the conversation. Her father was not an issue. He was not the suspect.

"Liquor. Mostly liquor. I distribute liquor. All over the Chicago area."

"What else?"

"What do ya' mean?"

"You said 'mostly.' What's the rest?" she asked.

"A little of this. A little of that. A couple of hockshops. Nothin' too big."

Or too legit. Al Capone had said it best. "Nobody's on the legit."

"If I'd had that done, it wouldn't have been done with a butcher knife. You can bet on that. Bullets. Real bullets. Nice dum-dums. He'd have had a set of holes that would have made his head look like a bowling ball. And he'd be someplace. Not left in his office. Or maybe he'd have been found in a car trunk at O'Hare. When the body started to smell."

He was certainly playing the role of somebody who wasn't on the legit. But was he on the legit? Was this just an act? Or was he coming clean with Donald Cater's little girl? Had her dad also not been on the legit? In that way? Did that make them family? She didn't want to be part of his family. The thought made her feel very queasy. And he thought her brother was a creep. If so, he was just a bush-league creep. Minor peccadilloes.

"I didn't kill John Doran. You have my sacred word for that."

And his word, she supposed, was his bond. Although he didn't say that it was. Thank God he spared her that one.

"And I didn't lay a hand on my daughter. Correction, my stepdaughter. Did I, honey?"

"No," Mrs. Kroller intoned. The statue could talk. It could probably even move.

"Of course, now he can't testify," Kroller mused. "Against me. Or against anyone else."

Kroller was now focusing his glare on his wife. What a pair! Not beauty and the beast. She did have a beauty to her. Like Marlene Dietrich. A cold, harsh beauty. But he was handsome. Rugged, strong. All he had to do was keep his mouth shut and he looked like a well-preserved athlete. A bit weathered, but all the sexier for it. It was more the reserved and the uncouth. Ice woman and caveman. The fastidious and the earthy. Had they ever been lovers? Not in years, she'd bet.

"Did you, honey?"

"Did I what?" Mrs. Kroller inquired.

"Kill John Doran."

"Of course not."

"I'd believe her. She hasn't touched a butcher knife since we got married. And she hasn't made love in even longer."

"William!"

"Or did you help me do it with dear sweet little Leslie? So I wouldn't bother you?"

"Really." The statue almost seemed angry.

"It never happened." He had shifted his attention back to Dennie now. "I never touched that little girl. I loved her. I worshipped her. She was my little angel. Believe me." He got up. He was standing at the window, looking out. "She grew up in this house. We used to play on that beach. She'd bury me in the sand." His nostalgia turned to anger. "It is time for you to go, Ms. Cater." He all but spit out her name. "I'll walk you to your car." He got up, walked over to the chair that held her coat, picked it up and held it for her. Their meeting was over.

As she struggled into her 'vette, she saw him staring up her thighs. He was a dirty old man. Instead of yanking her skirt down, she let it pull up an inch farther by letting her left leg fall farther toward the left.

He knew she'd done that on purpose.

"Smoking cigars isn't the only thing I've had to give up," he said, looking away.

"Your wife?"

"Screw her!"

"That's what I meant."

"I was telling the truth in there. About her, at least. The Ice Princess."

"Then why. . . ?" She didn't have to finish the question.

"It was her dad's business. Pizzetti. Pizzetti and Sons. The old man had four sons. Four dead sons. All shot. One in the Korean War. He's the only one who died slowly. It was all business," he went on. "We're business partners. That's all it's ever been. Did Gilbert like Sullivan?"

He hadn't.

"It's other women I've had to give up."

"I'm sorry."

"I had a good run. I've got maybe six months left. Maybe a year. But now maybe I'll be able to die in peace."

"Now?"

"With that bum Doran dead, the trial will get set back until I'm dead."

"That makes his death pretty convenient for you."

"Life is full of convenient surprises. Sometimes, at least. Thanks for the view. It brought back some good memories. Your dad was a good guy. More on the legit than me. And luckier to have daughters like you. Lucky guy. I wish I had my little girl back."

There was nothing she could say.

"Keep your nose clean."

With that he turned and walked back into his house.

She wanted to believe him. To believe that he was innocent. That he was on the legit in this one. And she still wanted to believe her dad had been innocent, too. Jack Kennedy had probably believed his old man was on the legit. Fantasies sometimes were hard to suppress.

She looked back at the house. The door was open. The black bodyguard was filling up the doorway. He smiled at her. His smile was terrifying. He could slip a knife into someone's chest without half an effort. Just to spare his boss some aggravation. Like killing a fly. A mere peccadillo.

As soon as she started driving, the nausea began to build up again in the back of her throat. She was no stranger to this feeling. She had been fighting off such episodes since she'd been a little girl. Even the chills were easier to take. The nausea was the worst. It made her feel even more frightened. More anxious. It was more than a sensation. It had a physical presence. Filling her whole mouth. All the way to the back of her throat. One more millimeter back and she would be gagging. She focused on it. On the sensation. Just on the sensation. And as she did, she gained control. It began to recede. Slowly. Millimeter by millimeter. Not backwards down her throat. She had to prevent that. Forward. It had to be pushed out. Over her tongue. Between her teeth. Through her open lips. Panting helped. There, it was leaving. It was out. Where it belonged.

※※※※

Dennie heard the alarm go off. She was not fully asleep. She'd slept for only a few minutes. Each time she drifted off, she awoke. Sick to her stomach. Gagging. Except the sensation was not in her stomach. Kroller. All he had done was touch her. He probably thought he had merely touched poor Leslie. Why was she so afraid of him? He wasn't going to touch her. Not in that way. So damn afraid.

Had he killed Doran?

Did he want to kill Beth?

And her?

And he had touched her. Defiled her. Polluted her. All the perfumes of Arabia. . . . UGH! So she'd been half awake–half asleep, waiting for the alarm to go off. And thinking about William Kroller. He was dying. Of what? Cancer? Heart disease? Either of them was likely. Served him right. He was a heavy smoker. Like her dad had been. Nausea. In the back of her throat. Pant. That always helped. It hadn't been this bad in years.

Too much like her dad. Too damn much.

The alarm was still buzzing at her. It was time for her to get up. It was almost five. The reception started at five-thirty. She knew that it was fashionable to arrive late. With the in crowd. The movers and the shakers. The people who were giving all those millions to help build the new Museum of Contemporary Art. Not her cup of tea, thank you.

What to wear? The eternal question. Black. She looked good in black. How she might look was irrelevant.

Basic black. Black pants, a black blouse. Silk. With one bright pin. The one she'd bought in Paris last year. That everyone thought was a Calder. It wasn't. Those bright splashes of color along the snail-like shape were more out of Niki de Saint Phalle than Calder. And matching earrings. And a leather jacket. Perfect. And dark enough.

She took a cab to the MCA. There was a small crowd gathered in the lobby. Most people seemed as if they were waiting for a funeral, not an art opening. Basic black was in. Damn. She should have worn something else. Fire engine red. Shocking pink. See-through net. No, someone else was wearing that. A see-through black net.

No one was saying anything except for one couple. And they were far too animated. And too loud.

"I hate art that I have to read," he complained vigorously. "It's no longer art. It's literature. It's a comic book." He was bald, just under six feet tall, thirty pounds overweight, and about fifty. A very vigorous fifty. And perhaps more than thirty pounds overweight. And he spoke far too damn loudly. Was he lecturing?

"Shush," the woman responded. She was ten years younger, eight inches shorter, and not a pound overweight. She looked elegant in her basic black. As refined as Mrs. Kroller wanted to be, but alive. Not cold at all.

"It's like those movies you have to read. They aren't movies. They are films." He pronounced the word 'fillems' as in 'fill-em-up.' "I hate them, too. Nobody likes those foreign fillems. Except foreigners who don't have to read them."

"You hate every movie since *Casablanca*," she reminded him.

"That's not true. I like *The Third Man*."

"That's what I meant," she smiled at him. She must have been through this argument more than once. And Dennie doubted that she'd ever lost.

"Art you have to read. Is that supposed to be conceptual?"

She ignored this remark completely. Her failure to reply seemed to invigorate him to a higher level of intensity. "You know what I like about conceptual art?"

"What? I thought you hated conceptual art."

"I do. But what I like," he continued, ignoring his own self-contradiction, "is that all you have to do is think about buying it and you're done. That saves me money."

She again said nothing.

"Get it?"

"I got it."

"You see if it's conceptual, then the concept of buying it should be sufficient."

"I got it," she reminded him.

The inside door leading into the museum itself opened. "Oh boy," he said. "Now I get to read some art." He dashed in, leaving her to trail in after him. She didn't. She walked in as if she were alone. Or if not alone, totally self-sufficient. Dennie was willing to bet that she was.

Dennie followed her in. The reception was in the gallery to the right of the entrance. The gallery was about half the size of the Kroller's living room. About fifteen by thirty-five. With a fifteen-foot ceiling and no chandelier. The reception was in honor of the first one-person museum show for a young Chicago artist named Libby Wadsworth. It was her pictures that filled the gallery. About twenty of them.

And he was right. That clod. You did have to read the pictures. That was not exactly her cup of tea either. Dennie planted herself in front of one of them. It was reminiscent of a cubist still life. Out of Braque. Out of Picasso. Out of that period when it was hard to tell where Picasso ended and Braque began. Not fully analytical. Lots of browns. Some well-defined shapes. A hint of Juan Gris. And with a diagrammed sentence working its way in and out. A sentence right out of Gertrude Stein. A perfect blending of the verbal and the visual. The reconstruction of words and images.

She loved it. She loved seeing it. Reading it. Getting inside of it. Stepping back and staying outside of it.

The next one was totally different. Yet more the same than seemed possible. Not in browns but in grays. Not cubist but looser. More out of an unfinished Cézanne still life. Or a Renoir. One gray apple. Had Cézanne ever painted a gray apple? Had Renoir? Could either of them? That gray. It reminded her of some other painter. But who? She knew. Giacometti. Not his sculptures, his oils. His gray oils. An apple out of Cézanne, by way of Giacometti. And again there was a single sentence. "It could have been but it doesn't seem likely." Not diagrammed, but surrounding the apple which was, of course, an image of an apple as Cézanne might have seen it. The sentence enveloped the apple. Making it an image. A device. A real image of an image.

"I own that one," a voice said.

She turned. It was Tom Ward.

"I bought it before she had a gallery to represent her. It's cheaper that way."

"Great insight."

"Luck," he chuckled. "I don't tell people about the ones I bought from nobodies who never became has-beens, because they have never been. I've got a room full of them. I'll show them to you someday."

"Are you asking me up to your apartment?"

"No. Not at all," he answered quickly.

"Too bad," she said. "It was a nice variation. Paintings instead of etchings."

"I have etchings, too," he said.

"Too late."

They shared the rest of the exhibit. Ambling together from picture to picture. Meandering back and forth. Crisscrossing the gallery. Looking at one and then back to another one and taking plenty of time to read each of them. To study each. At least once. Up close. From reading distance. Then from farther away, from picture distance. It was the best show she'd seen in a Chicago museum since the Art Institute had housed the Paschke show. And she'd seen that show in Paris. She wanted very much to see Tom's room of rejects. And his collection. Even his etchings

When they got to the last picture, he was there. The bore. She cringed. At least he had stopped pontificating.

"Hi, doc," Tom said.

Doc! Tom knew this jerk. He was a doctor. What else? Some overbearing surgeon who was worried that the government might decrease his earnings to a low seven figures. Pompous ass.

"Tom," the bore said with a nod and then, not even allowing time for a brief introduction, he surged on. "What a brilliant show. One part Braque, one part Picasso. More Braque than Picasso. With a hint of Gris. A touch of Cézanne. A pinch of Stein. Gertrude not Leo. And more than a whiff of Apollinaire. One must never forget Apollinaire. To say nothing of Max Jacob. I suppose you already own one."

"I do."

"Someday I'll find an artist before you do. Or, more likely, my wife will. She made me come tonight. I don't know where I'd be without her."

"I'll bet you told her that you hated art you have to read," Tom said.

"You got it," he replied laughingly. "And the funny part is that I still do."

"You missed one," Dennie said.

"One what?" Richardson asked.

"One of her influences," she said.

"I did. Who did I miss?"

"Giacometti."

"You're right. His oils. Tom, who is this bright, beautiful blond?"

She was pleased that *bright* came first.

"Professor Richardson, this is Dennie Cater," Tom then said.

The two of them shook hands.

"Doc is a neurologist. A professor at Austin Flint. A brilliant guy. He's an expert on Huntington's disease. In fact, he once wrote an article about witchcraft in Salem. You did, didn't you, doc?"

"Yes."

"Dennie's interested in witchcraft."

"Call me," he said. "I'll be happy to help you. Any friend of Tom's. I've got to go. My wife is about to buy one of these and I'd like to get my two cents worth in if she'll let me."

He started to walk away, then turned to her. "My wife loves Niki de Saint Phalle. Where did you get those earrings?"

"Paris."

"But where in Paris?"

"Rue des Saints Pères. Right next to Hotel des Saints Pères."

"Thank you. And do call. I don't bite. In fact, I'm perfectly harmless."

She doubted that.

"Tom," he added, "this one is a winner. Don't screw it up."

✳✳✳✳

If the Kroller's house was out of Margaret Mitchell, the late John Doran's office was out of a Roger Brown painting. And Dennie knew exactly which painting. The one in Sean Keneally's conference room. With its never-ending succession of strip malls. All that was missing was a K-Mart. Or a Wal-Mart. Or some other sort of mart. Doran's office was in one of the more nondescript strip malls on Clybourne, a diagonal street cutting through much of the northern half of Chicago. Once a proud industrial street, it was now home to a succession of such nondescript malls. Each one seemingly more nondescript than the prior one, no matter which direction you were coming from. Or was it less nondescript. That one she'd have to ask Beth.

There were only about half a dozen cars in the parking lot. And all of them were congregated at the northern end outside some pancake outlet that claimed that it was the original such pancake emporium, not to be confused with any other identically named original pancake restaurant. There had, she recalled, been three original Alfredo's in Rome. Each one less authentic than the other two, if her memory served her well.

She parked her 'vette near the southern end of the lot. She was beginning to like that car. This end of the mall was very dark. She was certain she'd be hard to see, all dressed in black. None of the businesses at that end were still open. It was after eleven. She had planned it that way. Not the quick copy franchise. Not the video store. Not the greeting card store. Nor Doran's office. Strips of bright yellow tape crisscrossed the door front, proclaiming it to be some sort of police secure zone and off limits to everyone. It didn't say positively.

Dennie reached into her purse as she got out of the car and retrieved her keys, including the keys that Beth had sent her. She fingered the keys until she had the right one ready.

Go.

A quick jog to the doorway. A black-clad figure in a dark parking lot. She felt like a character in a B movie. The kind of movie that Paul Richardson probably loved. And that his wife tolerated for him.

She inserted the key into the lock. And turned it. It turned. Would wonders never cease? And the door swung open. She withdrew the key, dropped it back into her purse and stepped through the crisscrossed tape. She was in. She closed the door behind her. Nothing to it. Now all she had to do was stop shaking like a leaf. And have her heart stop pounding. She took her pulse. 140. Why was she so damn frightened? No nausea, she commanded herself. She was like a scared little girl. But she wasn't a helpless little girl anymore. She was in control of her body now.

She took two deep breaths. Then another half dozen. Not quite as deep. Her pulse slowed to a mere 120. She was winning.

Where to look? Where to start? Where Beth had told her to look. Where else? The alcove behind John Doran's desk.

She shoved the door open and turned on the light. It was not an ordinary alcove. It was more of a cross between a video outlet store and a library. Shelf after shelf filled with videotapes. All numbered. Consecutively. And labeled with coded labels. Labels made up of a mixture of numbers and letters. Each digit could be either a number or a letter. Like a license plate.

She had no idea what the code meant. And no idea how to figure it out. And no desire to make the effort.

She wanted the most recent tapes. But which ones were the recent ones? Were the tapes filed chronologically? Alphabetically? By patient? By diagnosis? By code number? She was no decoder.

The shelved tapes gave no hint as to which tapes were recent and which were old. At least not that Dennie could tell.

Perhaps he had a code book in his office. She turned and as she did, the outer door flew open. A cold wind blew into the office. Once again she started to shake. And her heart began to pound.

And, she remembered, no one else was even parked within a hundred feet.

A big male shape filled the doorway. A big black male. As big as Kroller's black bodyguard. And just as black. Shit. That Kroller bastard.

Eller, that was his name. She knew she couldn't trust Kroller. He was capable of doing anything to her. Of ordering Eller to do anything. A heart attack was too good for him.

How big was a Corvette's trunk? Would she fit inside? How long would it take before anyone missed her? Jessie was away. Beth was on the lam. Tom Ward could hardly be expected to notice.

Damn it. Get it over with. Wait! It wasn't Eller. This dude had hair. Not much, but some.

That was better. Or was it even worse? This guy looked like he knew Godzilla, personally. He had a flashlight. It was more like a torch than a flashlight. Whatever it was, he pointed it directly into her eyes, making her blink and squint. And look away.

"You lost, ma'am?" the voice said.

"Police business," she said.

"I'm the police," he said.

"Thank God," she said.

"And you're breaking and entering. More like broke and entered."

"Sheriff's office," she said. "I'm here to check this guy's state and county licenses."

"You wouldn't happen to have your badge, would you?"

"I sure do," she said. She fished into her purse. Hoping it was there. It was. She flashed the badge her father had had in the old days of politically appointed deputy sheriffs. It even had her name on it. "D. Cater."

"Well, you look around all you want to, but you can't remove anything."

"You mean because of the murder investigation?"

"I mean because of the restraining order!"

"Restraining order? I don't get it."

"One of his patients went and got a restraining order. Something about privileged communication. Doctor-patient shit. It's beyond me. All I know is that you can't take nothing. You can't even listen to the tapes. But feel free to look all around. Good night, ma'am."

"Good night," she replied.

The door closed.

Take nothing. Listen to nothing. Look all around. She did. She didn't find a code book. Or an appointment book. She once again saw all of his diplomas. Including a couple from someplace called the Jung Institute of Chicago. Not exactly the University of Chicago.

And some videotapes. Not many. There were four unlabeled tapes on the desk. Just sitting there. Invitingly. Were they new or used?

She looked at them closely, They'd been used. And they had not been rewound. She walked slowly back into the alcove and pulled out a tape. It had been rewound.

Another. Also rewound.

A third. Ditto.

And a fourth. Of course.

Bingo. Four recently used tapes. Never rewound. Sitting there and waiting to be viewed. The restraining order, she assumed, did not apply to her. She wasn't a cop. She'd gotten in illegally. She picked up the four tapes, slid them under her leather jacket, and left, locking the door behind her.

"Good night, ma'am," came a voice from the shadows. She almost jumped out of her skin.

"Did you find what you needed?"

"Yes."

"But you didn't take nothing?"

"Of course not. The restraining order."

"Good. Then I don't have to list you on my report."

It was only after she had driven out of the lot that she realized that he had never shown her his badge. And after she'd shown him hers. Not exactly fair.

Chapter
V

Dennie needed to go to sleep. And not to dream. If it were only a slim perchance. That was wrong. *Perchance* wasn't a noun. No matter, it still rubbed her the wrong way. Kroller had murdered sleep. Or had he? Someone had? Who? And when? And how and why?

She tossed and turned and finally sleep came. Then she was no longer alone. Someone was in her room. A man. Above her. Coming down toward her. Closer. Ever closer. He was big. So damn big. Too damn big. Nausea. Filling her mouth. Her throat. Gagging her. She was going to gag. To vomit. She awoke. Sweating. Panting. Swallowing hard.

She turned on the lights. No one was there. She turned on her TV. And she watched. Reruns of old shows she never watched when they were the ones to be watched. And dozed off between ads. A few minutes at a time.

At a little after six, Dennie decided to have breakfast in bed. Not that she had that much of a breakfast. Some hot coffee, a glass of orange juice. She took both of them into her bedroom. She had four videotapes to choose from. She'd wanted to watch them as soon as she'd gotten home, but she'd been too tired. And too frazzled. Now she was just frazzled. If she were going to help Beth, she had to be in far better control of herself. Easier said than done. She was no detective. She had no idea how to solve a murder. Murder scared her. All violence did. Concentrate! She had to concentrate. She started by rewinding the four tapes. Which one should she watch? How could she tell? She couldn't. They weren't listed in *TV Guide,* which she never read.

She slipped the top tape into her VCR, propped all her pillows up in one place in the bed, on the left side next to the nightstand, got back in under the covers, took a couple more sips of coffee, and pushed POWER and then PLAY on her remote. The TV switched on.

Taking the four videotapes had been so damn easy. Perhaps too damn easy. Even with that cop there. It had almost been as if the police had wanted her to take the tapes. Perhaps they did. They couldn't take them themselves. They were restrained from that. By a restraining order. But that restraining undoubtedly had its own restraints. Its own limitations. It could only apply to videos found in John Doran's office. And contiguous places. Well, her apartment wasn't contiguous with his office. Not by a long shot. And the tapes were unmarked.

All in all, that was an interesting possibility. Perhaps that scenario was a bit too subtle. These were the Chicago cops. Subtlety was not their strong point. Strong arms were. Did Tom Ward have strong arms? He was certainly capable of subtlety.

Who had gotten that restraining order? A patient, supposedly. According to that cop. The one who hadn't shown her any ID.

Which patient? Undoubtedly, a patient with clout. Dennie could think of one such patient. Leslie English. She had clout. Sean's clout. Clout of the highest order. Mainline Irish Democratic clout. Democracy at work. Chicago style. Like hot dogs and pizza. Only better. And there were other people in this town with clout. Lots of them. It didn't have to be Sean.

Did it matter? She had the videos. Four unlabeled videos. That looked like any other videos. And she had them in her apartment. And no one was restrained from taking her videos. Or from watching them. Not even the cops. They could take them from her. All they had to do was get a search warrant for Beth's and remove the contiguous tapes. All four of the tapes had been sitting there in a single pile. Sticking out like a sore thumb. Almost as subtle as those potions in Wonderland. But instead of a placard saying "eat me," the tapes all but had a sign saying "take me." The TV screen flashed on.

And on it was the image of the couch in John Doran's office. This time the couch was empty. There was no naked body on it. No butcher knife coming out at a sixty degree angle. No pool of dark red blood. Just a couch with no one on it. Living or dead. Hardly sinister. Watching the empty couch was almost as boring as watching a cricket match on the BBC. More men standing around playing with their own bats.

Whoops, something was happening.

A number appeared on the screen. Near the top. Toward the left. The number 2 had moved toward the right. Almost all the way to the center of the screen.

Then came a hyphen.

Then two digits: 1 and 2. 12.

Another hyphen and then the rest of the date. 2-12-93. The date centered itself at the top of the screen. 2-12-93. That was the date of John Doran's death. She'd picked a good tape. She hadn't picked that tape. Someone else had. And that someone had picked a good tape. Who?

And why?

And for whom?

This sure had cricket beat. It was right up there with snooker. Watching the guys rub chalk on the end of their cues.

So this was what Doran did between patients. She'd often wondered what shrinks did in the ten minutes between patients. Doran made his own titles, with the computer at his desk. Jessie would know just how he did that.

Another line was taking shape. This one started with numbers.

It was the time. The time of the videotape. The time of the appointment. The session. 6:00 P.M. On the evening of the murder.

She'd picked a very good tape. Doran had gotten himself killed at around ten. If only it turned out to be a four-hour tape.

Then came a series of letters.

Please use the whole name. Not some code.

JOHN

John what?

JOHN JOHN

That Kennedy kid?

JOHN JOHNSTON

Not the Kennedy kid, but a patient named John Johnston. That was the name of the patient John Doran had seen at 6 P.M. on the evening he'd been stabbed. On 2-12-93.

Some more letters popped up. On the next line. And became a word. SESSION.

And then a second word: NUMBER

SESSION NUMBER 19.

This had been John Johnston's nineteenth session with John Doran. That meant that he was not a new patient. He'd been his patient long enough to have had eighteen previous sessions. And eighteen other videos filed away somewhere in that alcove behind Doran's desk.

Now it was time to see the patient.

"Come in, John," an off-camera voice said. That was John Doran's voice. Dennie recognized it.

"Hello, Dr. Doran," another voice said, also off-camera.

He wasn't a doctor.

"Mister," Doran reminded his client.

The other voice said nothing.

A door closed.

And a man lay down on the couch. What a hunk. Mid to late twenties. Six foot. Curly brown hair. Dark eyes. He wore tan slacks and a white shirt, open at the neck. Two buttons had been left unbuttoned. Why not three? Or four?

The shirt was cut very narrow. And so was John Johnston. Richard Gere had very little on this guy.

"How are you, Doctor?" he asked.

"I'm good, John. And you?"

"Okay, I guess."

"You're more than okay," Dennie said, reaching for some orange juice. He, of course, made no reply to her. Life was like that most of the time. Her life.

"Shall we get started?"

John Johnston stretched out and folded his hands behind his neck. He licked his lips. Once. Twice. "I did it again," he said.

Doran uttered a noncommittal "yes."

She recognized the technique from when she'd studied psych. It had been called nondirective therapy. À la Adler. Having been a psychology major wasn't entirely useless. Just almost so.

"Twice. I know I promised you I'd stop," the patient said, his eyes half closed.

That didn't sound nondirective to her. The patients of nondirective therapists didn't make promises to their therapists.

"I thought we had a deal," Doran's voice said, firmly and harshly and with more than a trace of disappointment in it.

"I didn't place a new ad. I didn't do that. I wouldn't break my promise to you." John sounded desperate.

"What happened?" Doran asked.

You couldn't get more directive than that.

"A John called me."

"Who?"

"Does it matter?"

Of course.

"Probably not."

"His name was John. That's all I know."

A plethora of Johns. This was more fun than any of the soaps. John Johnston. John Doran. And John. John Doe. Too many Johns. Christ, she realized with a shock of recognition, this John Doe was a John. John the John. Both in name and function. Much better than the soaps.

"And. . . ," John Doran prompted his client.

"He'd seen my personal ad. You know the one. The old one."

Doran obviously did.

"So I went to his place and gave him a massage. It was no big deal."

"You call giving him a massage no big deal."

"Yeah," defiantly. "No big deal."

What was the big deal? A massage was a massage. All massages were equal.

"And he was naked?"

"Yes," still defiant.

"And so were you?"

"Yes," no longer as defiant.

And not so equal either.

"And you gave him a full body massage?"

"Yes," not defiant at all.

"And what did he do?"

John Johnston had tears in his eyes.

"I asked you a question," the therapist reminded him.

The patient said nothing. He was sobbing now.

"John. What did this man do to you? Tell me."

"He gave me a massage."

"And he paid you?"

"Of course."

"How did that make you feel?"

"Shitty."

"Tell me about your father again."

The transition threw Dennie for a loop. What did his father have to do with all of this? She could feel her body tensing.

John Johnston understood. "That cold SOB," he responded.

That description and that interchange typified the next twenty minutes of session number nineteen. Like a dentist on a holy quest, John Doran probed. And probed. And probed again. Until he got pain. Until John Johnston winced. Until he cried out in pain. Then onto another tooth. More probing. Then back to the sensitive spot. And probing at it again. And again. And then pain. More pain.

And the most sensitive spot was John Johnston's father. His cold, aloof, stern father. A patriarch among patriarchs. Distant. Frigid. Unable to show approval. Unable to show any affection at all. Any love.

Then a shift. Very abruptly. Instituted once again by the therapist. "Tell me about your dreams."

"I don't dream," John argued. "I've told you that before."

"We all dream," Doran said.

"But we don't all remember them," John said.

"We all can remember them with the right help."

"So help me."

A stalemate. Of sorts. Neither voice said anything for almost a minute. It was like a TV time-out for a commercial except this time the director forgot to cut away from the sight of inactivity. Dennie took two more sips of her coffee.

It had cooled off so she killed off the orange juice. Her analogy was wrong. She was eavesdropping on a war of nerves between two skilled combatants and this time the patient won. Wrong again. The client. The client had won. So the therapist was regrouping.

"Tell me about the dream about the fire. The one we were talking about last time." He had regrouped and come out fighting.

"I don't remember that dream. I didn't before."

The probe had been rebuffed.

"You will next time."

Another pregnant pause. A twenty-second time-out this time. The coffee was far too cold to sip.

"No more massages," Doran said. "That is not the way to get back at your father. Or to receive his affection."

John Johnston's face was expressionless. He was looking straight up at the ceiling of glass, at the window and the unseen camera, with a cold hard stare. Was that the look he had learned from his father?

"No more, I said."

"No more," the patient intoned. He did not sound convinced. Or convincing.

"Good. It's a deal. We don't want your father to find out."

"How could he?"

"I can think of two ways, at least. He might see your old ad and read it."

"Who keeps old *Readers?*" he asked. He was still staring at the ceiling. Right up at the camera. His expression was showing a touch of curiosity. Then a frown.

"Lots of people," Doran said.

"And who reads old ads?"

"More people than ever answer them."

"Not my father. He doesn't know sex exists." His expression was bordering on a glare.

"Where did you come from?"

"His one mistake."

"And he knows you're coming here."

"No. He doesn't. No one does. I pay my own bills. With cash. And even if he did, he doesn't have the right to see my records. And you told me you don't keep any notes. No written record at all." He was angry now. He jumped up. All she could see now was the top of his head. "You liar."

"I didn't lie to you."

"Then there are no records?"

"I take no notes. I don't write anything down," the therapist reassured him.

"So it couldn't make any difference, could it? Even if one of his goons broke in here, you never write anything down, right?"

"Right!"

"Keep it that way, Doctor."

"Our time is up."

John left the screen.

"See you next week," John the patient said.

"Same time," John the therapist reminded him. The door opened and closed.

Back to the empty couch.

PAUSE.

Dennie picked up her mug and went into the kitchen. She poured out the cold coffee and then poured herself a fresh cup of hot coffee. She opened the refrigerator, took out the milk. Two percent. And poured a small amount into her mug. Two percent of two percent. How much was that? Only Jessie could do that kind of higher math. Point 0–4 parts per hundred. Something like that.

Dennie had watched one hour of one tape and she already had another suspect. John Johnston. Especially if he'd figured out what was behind that small window. Sure, Doran didn't keep written records. He hadn't really lied. Why write out notes? He had videotapes of everything.

But at six forty-five on the evening of the murder, John Johnston didn't know that there was a camera in the ceiling. When he stared up at that ceiling of glass, he was curious. Then wondering. Then angry. Did he know? Did he figure it out? At that instant.

He certainly got angry. Pissed off. No question about that. Hell, being a detective might be fun. If all she had to do was watch videos. Somehow she knew that wouldn't be the case.

Dennie climbed back into her bed, cradled her mug on her chest, and pushed REWIND.

PLAY.

She'd gone too far. FAST FORWARD. There. This was the place. Doran was probing away. Causing pain.

FAST FORWARD.

PLAY.

Back and forth. Then she was there. "Where did you come from?"

She watched.

John Johnston was staring right at the camera. That meant he was staring at the glass window. He might have figured it out. Right then.

But was he angry enough?

He was.

She definitely had another suspect. Two had become three. Or four. ". . . even if one of his goons. . . ."

One of his goons. His father had goons. What sort of goons? What sort of goons were there? Only one sort that she could think of. And William Kroller didn't have a monopoly on all the goons in Chicago.

She had added two suspects in an hour. At this rate she'd soon have too many. She had been so absorbed that she hadn't once felt nauseated. Or frightened. Or even that anxious. Perhaps she was in better control of herself. If only it would last. The tape was back to the empty couch.

She was hungry. It was time for a little something, but what? All she had were some stale English muffins. She felt like something more continental. Fresh warm croissants that she could dip into her coffee.

Dennie turned off the VCR, got up, and pulled on yet another of her non-matching sweat suits. A Columbia sweat shirt and a pair of Northwestern sweat pants. The next time the three of them got together they'd have to trade sweat shirts and sweat pants so that she had at least one matching set. When? Or if? That possibility sent a chill through her. When? That was a far better question.

And she now had four suspects to work on. John Johnston, male masseur. That was a redundancy but it made the point. His father. Of goon fame. Leslie's mother. AKA Mrs. Kroller. And William Kroller. Dennie despised him. And was so damn afraid of him. He revolted her. A revulsion that hit her right in the guts. She needed him to be the one. To be caught. And convicted. And punished. For murder. And for molesting Leslie. And for. . . . Not every child molester was also a murderer. Just this one. She was feeling that nausea again.

Her phone rang. She jolted up in bed. Who? It was a double ring. Someone was buzzing her from downstairs. She grabbed the remote. On went the TV. She anxiously switched it over to channel 14. Who was there?

The lobby of her building came slowly into view. Why was it taking so damn long? As the image of the lobby sharpened so did the figure of Tom Ward, pressing a button next to the mail boxes.

She picked up the phone as it began to ring again.

"Hello, Tom."

"How did you know?" He stopped himself and waved at the camera.

Why not? That camera wasn't hidden from view. It wasn't behind any window. John Johnston had not waved at the camera.

"Hi," he said. "What are you doing?"

"What should a girl be doing on a Sunday morning? I'm laying in bed, thinking about breakfast," she lied, fighting for control.

"You're lying."

"I am not!"

"The correct tense for having your own body in a resting position in bed is lying. Laying in the present tense in relation to a woman and a bed has a far different connotation."

"I'm not laying," she said.

"Can I come up?"

"It depends on the connotation," she said. She hoped her banter was replete with self-assurance. If only he knew.

"I brought croissants."

"In that case any connotation at all is perfectly okay by me," she said as she pushed "6," heard the door buzz, and watched Tom Ward open it.

She only had half a minute or so.

EJECT.

The tape came out. She grabbed it and two of the other three and carried them into the living room. There was no time to label them so she just stuffed them in among her other tapes. The family vacation tapes.

She opened the door just as Tom got there.

"Great outfit," he said.

"I suppose you liked me better in my see-through nightgown?" Men!

"No."

"No?"

"Basic black. You looked great last night."

"Thank you."

He held up a white paper bag. "Croissants," he said.

"And not a moment too soon," she said, stepping back to let him in and then closing the door behind him.

They sat at the small table in her kitchen, sipping coffee and dunking their croissants. Ah, to be in Paris. Anytime. At least they were talking about art. Feeling each other out. Not probing. Just searching around.

He was single. Divorced. Why?

"She got tired of being a cop's wife."

Dennie wasn't sure she understood what that meant.

Long hours, he threw out as a starter.

So what? Lots of people had long hours.

Irregular hours.

That, too.

She had her own career.

And separate careers.

And her own interests.

And separate interests.

And they just grew apart. Too far apart. And she met someone. And when she told him, he felt relieved.

Clearly not a good sign.

They got divorced. Almost four years ago.

Children?

One. A son. Nineteen. In college. U.of I. Downstate. He missed him.

So much for the life and times of Tom Ward. By mutual consent they changed the subject to Dennie Cater and her life and times. She, too, was single. Never married. Never even engaged.

"Between engagements?" he asked.

"I said I was never engaged."

"I meant that in a theatrical sense. Actors are never unemployed. They're between engagements. I was trying to be polite."

"You're sweet."

"Not many people think that," he said.

"I do." Then she added, "and I am between engagements."

He took the last bite of his croissant.

"Does the name Kroller mean anything to you?" she asked, being less nondirective than John Doran at his worst.

"Yes."

"What?"

"He's well known in police circles. He's a liquor distributor, among other things."

"Such as."

"A couple of pawnshops. Some adult bookstores. Maybe even a legitimate front or two. Not too legit. Businesses with lots of cash flow. Dry cleaners. Food marts. That sort of thing."

"Mob ties?"

"What do you think?"

"Kroller's not an Italian name."

"Nor was Lansky. Besides Kroller isn't his real name. That was Cassotto. His father changed it to Kroller."

"Why?"

"He distributed liquor to Germans and Scandinavians. His first store was in the Andersonville area, up north."

"Johnston," she said. "That's another name."

"What is this, twenty questions?"

"Name that crook!"

"Why?"

"Just curious."

"Not a name I know."

She finished her last bite of croissant.

"Kroller's married to Leslie's mother. He had a kid by a previous marriage. Billie Junior. He's in the family business. Runs some of the video outlets. Officially that's what they're called. But Johnston," he then repeated, "that's not a name I recall."

"No children," she said changing the subject.

"No children?"

"Yes, I have no children."

"I didn't think that you had. You've never been married."

"I didn't know that that was still a prerequisite."

"I suppose it isn't. I guess I'm just old-fashioned."

"So am I," she agreed. "Sort of."

"I'll show you my tape," he said, "if you'll show me yours."

"What?" His change in the subject had caught her off guard.

"Your tape."

My tape. Did he mean Beth's tape? The tape of Beth and Doran's body. A tape that would place Beth at the murder scene with the dead body. Never. How did he know about that tape?

"We know you have one."

One?

"One what?"

"One tape. One of Doran's tapes."

"One of Doran's tapes?"

"Yes, the one you took from his office. Last night."

He didn't know about Beth's tape. Thank God. And he only thought she had one tape. How? That cop. Had he looked on the desk? Before and after her visit? But she took four videos, not one. Ward did know she'd taken something. Had she been set up? By him. This subtle but single cop.

"How do you know?" she asked.

"His secretary went into the office this morning. She thought that one of the tapes was missing. And you were observed last night."

"I took a tape," she confessed. One, not four. She had no idea what was on those other tapes. And she wanted to see them first. All by herself.

"I want to see it."

"Was I set up?"

"Would I do something like that?"

"I think I'll plead the Fifth on that one," she said. "But you have to show me yours first. Let's go into the bedroom." She blushed. She'd embarrassed herself. "That's where the VCR is."

He put his tape in and they sat on the foot of her bed. They were too close to the TV but it was less disconcerting that way.

His tape showed the couch. Doran's couch. The view from the ceiling.

"He had a very sophisticated set-up," Tom explained to her. "Still has. I mean the set-up is still there and fully functional. You recognize the couch, of course."

"Of course." Why lie? She was going to show him her tape.

"We modified it a bit."

She looked at him. She was tired of looking at that same couch.

"Now the camera goes on whenever someone enters his office and stays on until they leave."

"How?"

"You probably wouldn't understand. Sensors and things. Motion detectors."

He was probably right.

"Is this a tape of me?"

"Yes."

"I never went over to the couch."

"We have your voice."

"Turn if off."

He did. "Your turn," he said. "I want to see the tape you took."

"It's the one on the TV," she said.

He nodded, took his tape out of the VCR, and slipped Doran's tape in.

Who, she wondered, would be on this one? And why just one? Why hadn't she told him about all four of the tapes? There had been four of them there in Doran's office, all neatly stacked. Was she afraid that Beth was going to be on one of them? Beth! It could be this one. Dennie had to screen them first. Just to be certain that there was nothing about Beth. But who had left those tapes for her? All so neatly stacked? Beth? No. She could have taken them herself. She was there. She had those keys. The keys Beth gave to her. Damn. Damn. Damn. There were too many questions and too few answers.

2-12-93. Right day again.

3 P.M. Wrong time. Too early.

Leslie English. Wrong person. Not that wrong. At least it wasn't Beth. Session number 109.

"Do you mind if I lie back?" Tom asked.

"No, I'll join you. Lying that is."

Leslie and Doran exchanged brief salutations and in no time she was lying on the couch looking up at the ceiling.

Dennie and Tom were on her bed. Leslie was fully clothed. So were they. And all three were obviously uncomfortable.

And Leslie was also very angry. Very angry at John Doran. She wanted him to testify in her case against William Kroller. She always called him by his full name. William Kroller. Cold. Formal. Detached. Third person impersonal. Doran owed her that much. As her therapist.

He wouldn't do it. He never went to court. He would not testify for her. Why not? She needed his help.

His job was not to testify in court but to help her.

That would help her.

But not in getting better. They had a relationship. A therapeutic relationship. A bond. A very delicate bond. Lawyers could break that bond. She'd hear what he'd say in court. And the lawyers would twist his words. And her words. It would destroy all their hard work. He would not testify as her therapist. It would hurt her too much.

As an expert then!

An expert?

Her expert witness. Her expert witness on witchcraft.

No. He wouldn't. He wasn't an expert on witchcraft.

But he had other patients who had been through what she'd been through. Yes, he did. A number of them.

What number, Dennie wondered. Two, after all, was a number.

This could be for all of them, Leslie argued. Not just for her. But to help all of them. A landmark case. That was what Sean Keneally had told her it could be.

No.

Why not? That wouldn't violate their relationship. Or any of his relationships with his other patients.

He wouldn't. He didn't trust lawyers. Or judges. Or the system. He wanted to help her. He had helped her. She now knew the truth. That was how he would help her. And his other patients. That way. His way. And his only way.

"Leslie, we were talking about your dream."

"The twelve witches."

"And your mother."

"Mother makes thirteen."

"Relax. Think back. Concentrate. Concentrate on the witches. Think about them."

"I'm trying," she said, much more calm than she had just been.

"Keep trying. And keep relaxing. Think about the witches. The thirteen witches. The magic number. The coven. The coven of witches. The witches. Your witches. Relax."

"I'm getting there. I'm beginning to see them," Leslie said. "They are dancing. And they are dressed in black."

"That's good. Now focus in on them," John Doran instructed her. "Focus on their dresses. The long black dresses, and the dancing. Concentrate. They were dancing. The light was flickering. On their faces. The dancing faces. On their eyes. Dancing around the. . . ."

"Fire," she said, panting. "We were all dancing around the fire. The bonfire. At the base of our tree."

"Count them. Tell me exactly how many there are."

She counted ". . . nine, ten, eleven, twelve. A dozen. And my mother."

"That makes thirteen. A coven of witches. It's always thirteen. Thirteen is what makes it a coven. Do you remember any of their names?"

"Their names?" She hadn't tried to.

"The names of the witches. They had names. Remembering the names will help to destroy their power. Their magic. Once you have the names their hold will be broken."

She would try. She had to. To break their hold on her. To be free of them.

"Relax. Picture them. Name them."

She was trying. It wasn't easy. The names. The twelve names.

"Start with one."

"One name." That sounded easier. One name. It was coming. A name. It was almost there. It was. A name. "Collins, Mrs. Collins."

"Mistress Collins," Doran editorialized. "The first is often the hardest."

"Mrs. Weaver. Collins and Weaver."

The process went on and on. The names meant nothing to Dennie. She hardly listened to them. The last one sounded something like Berger.

"That's only twelve," he said.

"And my mother. Mother makes thirteen," she repeated.

"Next? What happened next?"

Her mother. Mom. Her mother was with her. Not just with her. She was holding her. Her mother was holding her. Holding her mouth open. Pouring in the blood.

Making her swallow the blood.

And then not letting her up.

Holding her.

Helping him take off her clothes.

Holding her.

For him.

For her stepfather.

For her father to. . . .

"It was her fault. Her fault. She forced me to do it," Leslie said.

"Yes," he said. "Our hour is over," he added.

Leslie got up and as she did the screen went blank for a moment.

"She amended her complaint to include her mother," Dennie said flatly.

"I know," Tom told her.

"That makes her mother a suspect."

"True. But can you imagine John Doran making love to her mother on his couch?"

She couldn't. Nor anyone else making love to Mrs. Kroller for that matter. Anywhere.

"And don't overlook your client."

"Leslie?"

"John Doran had scorned her."

That, too, was true, in a sense.

The image of the couch reappeared. And then another set of information began to form itself on the screen.

2-12-93

5 P.M.

Leslie had been there for two hours.

Robin Riegel.

Robin was young. Around twenty. She sat on the couch and exchanged small talk for several minutes. Some biographical data.

She was nineteen. A freshman at DePaul. That was not far from Doran's office. Less than a couple of miles. A very short bus ride.

She was from a small town in Wisconsin. A Catholic girl. At a Catholic college. Nothing strange about that.

Her mom had gone there. So had her dad. He'd been on the basketball team with George Mikan. He'd also taught there. That was how they'd met. His dad was older than her mom. About fifteen years older. Robin was beginning to relax.

The name Mikan obviously meant something to John Doran. And to Tom Ward, but not to her.

Robin was one of six children. The last one.

She lay down on the couch. Then it came out in a tumble. A torrent. Broken by sobs.

A date. With a senior. A basketball player. His name meant something to John Doran. And Tom Ward. Brian Havergal. It meant no more to her than George Mikan had.

Then back to her apartment. For coffee. Then he grabbed her. She tried to stop him. He was so big.

"Big Brian," Tom said.

"How do you know?"

"That's his nickname. He's the center. Almost as big as George Mikan was. In his day he was the biggest."

She tried to stop him. He was too big. She couldn't. She quit trying. She let him do it.

Twice.

She wanted to kill him. What could she do? She was so ashamed. Twice. She had let him do it again. She couldn't tell anyone. That SOB.

She was sobbing violently.

"You're not just angry at him." Doran said. The calm voice of a trained professional. He had heard all of this before.

"I hate myself. I'm so dirty."

"You couldn't have stopped him."

There was a pause.

"There is someone else you're angry at."

"There is."

"Yes."

"Who?"

"That is what we'll have to find out."

The session was over but you didn't have to be Sigmund Freud to figure it out. Or even Adler. Or Jung.

"He figures to be a first-round draft pick."

"Who?"

"Brian Havergal."

"So?"

"That's worth millions of dollars to him, unless he gets accused of rape. Then no NBA team would touch him."

"So?"

"We have one more suspect."

So they did.

"Do you have anything else to show me?" he asked.

"No. Do you have anything else to show me?"

He didn't.

"What about your etchings?"

"I don't show them professionally."

"I wasn't asking professionally."

It was almost two. He needed to check a few things at his office. He'd pick her up at four and they'd stay on neutral territory. The Chagall show at the Art Institute. And then dinner.

Chapter
VI

As she jogged along Dennie caught a brief line or two about the murder of John Doran on her jog-woman radio. There was not a word about any suspects. Or arrests. It was just another of Chicago's murders. One of the four they mentioned. One of the others was of a seven-year-old girl shot while waiting for a church bus. Wasn't life in the big city great? No wonder she was frightened and anxious so much of the time. Who wouldn't be?

Dennie had been jogging for about half an hour. It was time to call it quits. She had planned to run for longer, but it was cold and damp and her hair was getting too damn frizzy. She had a date. And she was getting too cold. One could only do so much for the sake of cardiovascular toning and good looks. It was only for the latter that she stuck it out as long as she did. She hated running, but they were going out for dinner. A brief stop for some juice and then home.

❋❋❋❋

There was a fax waiting for her in her apartment. Two, in fact. The first was from Beth. It wasn't addressed to her. The original had been sent from Beth to Sean Keneally. And, of course, signed *Elizabeth*. In it she retained Sean as her lawyer. Officially. She had sent him a retainer by separate cover. Probably a FedEx letter. A copy of the fax had been faxed to her. According to the time on the fax, it had been sent at the apex of her run. Or the nadir. That was a matter of perspective. Right in the middle.

Beth was obviously okay. And thinking about her future. And getting herself a lawyer. But why Sean? He was not a criminal lawyer. And nothing was more criminal than a murder charge.

Had she been charged? Officially? Not yet, at least not according to what Sean had told her. Maybe he didn't know everything. She could ask Tom Ward. It was his investigation. Why let a little thing like a murder charge in the family get in the way of romance? Was this romance? It was too early to tell. They were still in the sparring stage.

The second fax was addressed to her. It was from Sean, sent minutes later. Nearer the apogee. No, that she knew was wrong. As she had entered her final lap. She'd only done one lap. The homestretch.

It notified her that Sean was now representing Elizabeth and Three Sisters Limited, including all three sisters. Elizabeth, Denise, and Jessica. Due to that relationship, all interactions between Sean and the three sisters collectively and individually had become privileged communication. Undiscoverable. Whatever that meant. He assumed there would be no conflict of interest. That representing any one of the sisters and that sister's best interest would not be in conflict with the best interests of either of the other two.

He could bet on that.

If that situation arose, the four of them would have to resolve it, undoubtedly by naming co-counsels for the other two sisters. He doubted that that eventuality would ever arise.

So did she.

In the meantime, any interaction they had now or had had in the past was privileged.

So that was what it was called. Privileged communication. Jessica and Sean had had privileged communication. Why the hell was she so damn underprivileged?

Tom Ward arrived right on time. She liked that in a man. Or a woman. He also showed up without a means of transport. He'd been on duty. A squad car had dropped him off. She drove in her 'vette. He was impressed. More by her legs than by the car. Thank God. She was not interested in a man who was into penis envy in any of its various manifestations.

She parked in the underground lot downtown, just south of the Art Institute and he was polite enough to get out first, come around to her side of the 'vette, and help her out. And almost polite enough not to take advantage of the position to see even more of her thighs. Almost, but not quite. Almost was the most a girl could expect. Or wanted.

The Chagall show was small. The pieces weren't. They were huge. Enormous murals he had painted in Russia right after the Revolution to decorate the Jewish Theater. They were wonderful examples of classic early Chagall. Painted in that bygone era before he had evolved into creating a series of parodies of his own early masterpieces. Bright. Vibrant. Strong. Original. Meaningful. They'd been in storage in Russia for over sixty years. They had survived the Stalinist era. More than could be said for most of the writers who wrote for the Jewish Theater. And the directors. And the actors. And the audiences.

Once they were back in the car, Dennie asked him where he wanted to go.

"The Café Royale," he said. "My treat."

"I usually pay my own way on first dates."

"I'm old-fashioned," he reminded her.

"How old-fashioned?" she inquired.

"Very old-fashioned."

She was not quite sure what her question had really meant. Or his answer. But she knew exactly where the restaurant was. "I took a wine-tasting class in that building," she said. Someone had to say something. "With my dad. He was already . . . very sick. But it was something he wanted to do. We had a lot of fun. More fun that we'd ever had sharing anything else." Why had she brought that up. Why her father? Why now? When she had been so relaxed.

"It's the best English restaurant in town," he said.

"What?" she asked.

"I said it is the best English restaurant in town."

"Is that a condescending remark?"

"No. I really like it. But you're right. Most of the others seem to believe that the difference between lemon sole and Dover sole is that one is served with lemon."

"Isn't it?"

"No," he laughed, "they're different species of fish."

She shrugged.

Tom then went on to detail the differences. It was as if he were an expert on fish. Was he? She asked him.

No, he wasn't. A waiter at Wheeler's in London had told him the difference once. And he had remembered. That was at the original Wheeler's. On Compton Street.

She remembered Compton Street. With its sex shows. And peep shows. Hookers. Times Square. Only worse. Why even mention that street? Then they were there.

She gave the car to the doorman and they were ushered into a private alcove. Ordinarily it sat six, but it was set for two, seated next to each other.

"Very clever," she said.

"What?"

"A private room. This way no one can see what you're doing."

"I'm not going to do anything," he protested.

"That must be because you are out with a murder suspect's sister."

"That wasn't the reason. . . ," he tried to explain.

Then what was?

"I . . . we . . . if you really must know, I haven't been on a date in twenty years. And I figured I'd be less likely to embarrass us this way. Are you satisfied?"

She wasn't, she was embarrassed.

They ordered. Tom ordered veal for himself. She wanted the sole.

"Lemon or Dover?" the waiter asked. "The difference. . . ."

Dennie interrupted him and told him the differences between the two species. She, too, had listened and learned.

Tom studied the wine list. He ordered a Montrachet. That, she knew, had to be the most expensive white wine on the list.

In a moment the waiter was back, empty-handed. They did not have that year.

"May I?" she interrupted, taking the wine list. One quick look and she ordered. A Pinot Grigio.

The waiter smiled. "That is probably our best white wine, madame." It was better than ma'am.

Tom was impressed.

Thanks, dad.

The wine came. Then the appetizers. And small talk. The Chagall panels. His idea of installation art. Site-specific installation art.

She thought that site-specific installation art was a gallery full of broken pieces of stone, just enough to fill that specific space.

"Too minimalist," he said. Not his idea of great site-specific installation art.

"An oxymoron," she suggested.

"The Sistine Chapel," he countered.

She chuckled.

"The Elgin Marbles," assuming she knew that the Elgin Marbles were the sculptures from the Parthenon. Even in the British Museum, they were still very site-specific.

"Touché," she conceded, sipping her Pinot Grigio. The salads arrived and he changed the subject to music. He loved Philip Glass. She hated Philip Glass. Not disliked, but hated.

Did she really know Philip Glass? Had she really taken the time to listen to his music? To his "Songs from Liquid Days?"

No.

Then how could she hate him? How could she be such a Philistine?

No one had ever called her a Philistine before. Had he seen that minimalist one-woman show at Lockett's Gallery? A soft wall with a single vertical opening. Sort of a slit. With soft edges. That undulated open and shut. Open then shut. It was supposed to be a vagi. . . .

"I know what it was supposed to be," she cut him off.

The main course arrived. Along with another bottle of Pinot Grigio. The conversation turned from Glass songs, to Glass operas, to the Lyric Opera's production of his "Satyagraha," which she had missed, to this year's season and the new Ring Cycle. Opera was a very safe subject. Much safer than vaginal installations.

They passed on dessert. Instead they had some cheese. Stilton and double Gloucester. And finished off the Pinot Grigio.

"Who managed to get that restraining order?" she asked. Not exactly a subtle question. But sometimes you had to ask a direct question in order to get a direct answer.

"Your boss."

That was certainly a direct answer. "Sean?" He nodded. "I didn't know that."

"There's probably no reason why you should. He was acting on behalf of his client," Tom said.

"Leslie," she guessed. "Doran can't testify. Not his choice this time. Maybe the courts will let her tapes in as evidence. Evidence that can't be cross-examined. Pretty clever. Very clever."

"I told you she had a motive," the detective replied.

"I thought you said that motives didn't matter," Dennie countered.

"Sometimes they do."

"I see," she said, even though she didn't. "Did that bug you?"

"The restraining order? Not really. We deal with things like that all the time. They're pretty routine. This is the sort of thing I'm supposed to be good at," he added.

"And what's that?"

"Tricky cases. Ones involving people with political connections. That's my bag."

"Like the Krollers? And Sean?" she wondered aloud.

"And the Caters."

Dinner was over, Tom paid the bill. "Old-fashioned," he reminded her. Then he suggested that they go to his place.

Perhaps he was not so old-fashioned at that.

"I want to play some Philip Glass for you."

Or perhaps he was.

"And show you my etchings."

They both laughed, perhaps more than was called for. Only time would tell.

❋❋❋❋

Some of Tom's pictures were almost like old friends. One was a Ray Yoshida that had been shown in half a dozen museums and reproduced in a couple of art books. "Jizz and Jazz" was the title. So were a couple of early Wirsums. Two of them had been in the retrospective at the MCA.

She had loved that show. She had almost lived with it. It had been that summer. But she didn't go into the details with him.

He also had Roger Browns. Lithographs. And Paschkes. Etchings, not oils. And newer artists. Younger ones. Some she knew. Several she didn't. She wrote down the names. Donna Tadelman, David Russick. Richard Hull.

And throughout the tour, the CD of Philip Glass' "Songs from Liquid Days" was playing. The first song had something to do with a hum in the wall. The melody was fragmentary, repetitive, hypnotic. Dennie listened as carefully as she could.

"A drink?" he whispered, trying not to disturb her listening.

"Yes," she whispered back.

He got up from the couch and in a few bars was back, handing her a snifter with brandy in it. She suddenly realized that he was far less comfortable than she was.

"Is there any record of a fax?" she asked.

He wasn't sure what she meant.

If someone sent a fax from a machine in a store, like the one near her apartment.

"A local call?"

"Yes."

"Cash?"

"Yes," she assumed.

"No. The clerk wouldn't know who had made which call. And there'd be no way to tell."

"No, I mean the fax itself. Not the call."

"You really don't know?" He was surprised.

She really didn't.

"The fax doesn't exist. It's like a Xerox machine. You put in the document and out comes a copy. What's in the middle has no real existence. Only the hard copy, the one that comes out at the other end, only that really exists. Why?"

"I was just wondering," she lied, much relieved.

He played along and said nothing.

The first song was long over. The one that was now being sung had the same drive, but a richer orchestration and was about lightning.

Tom was now talking about the Krollers. He, too, thought that they were both suspects. That meant that he at least had not closed the case. His reasoning pretty much paralleled her own.

"Kroller could be very dangerous. He has important connections," he reminded her. As if she needed to be reminded. "He has dangerous connections."

"Political?"

"And otherwise." It was the "otherwise" that bothered him and should, he hoped, scare her.

It did, more than he realized.

"I want to make a deal with you," he added. "You ignore the Krollers. I'll work on that angle."

"And. . . ?"

"You check out the others."

"Meaning?"

"Big Brian."

She nodded her assent. He seemed far less threatening.

"And your client."

"Leslie?" She was surprised. Was Leslie really a suspect? That motive about the videotapes as being better for her case than a therapist who didn't want to get involved didn't sound too promising to her. But what did she know about motives? "Is Leslie really a suspect?"

"Everyone's a suspect."

"Even me?"

"No. Not you. Just those four, so far. Unless Johnston's a suspect."

"Who?" she asked, hoping he had not noticed how off guard she'd been caught. He'd gone fishing. And landed a nibble.

"Nothing," he said. "Just a name. For now."

They both understood. Some professional secrets could remain unshared for a little while. They both returned to listening to Philip Glass. Why was he sitting so far away from her, she wondered. Tom was clinging to his brandy snifter and sitting as far away from her as he could without getting off the couch they were both occupying and moving to the chair behind the desk.

"How long has it been?" she asked.

"Since Leslie has been a suspect?"

"No. I'm asking about you," she corrected him. "How long?"

"How long?" he echoed, hoping he had not understood her question. He knew he had.

So did she. "I'll spell it out. How long has it been since you made love to a woman?"

Tom took a deep breath. He would tell her. "Four years, almost."

He was nervous.

She was in control. Total control. And they both knew it. But neither of them was embarrassed. It was as if personal honesty were more important than any professional honesty.

"To anyone other than your wife?" she continued.

He knew he had to supply an answer. Some answer.

"Well?"

He could not just invent some answer. They both knew that.

"Since I got married," he replied, without calculating his answer.

"You're kidding," she said.

They were both quiet now. They remained seated on the same couch as far apart as two people could be while sharing the same piece of furniture. Had it been a sectional couch, she was sure that the forces that they were generating would have propelled the sections into opposite corners of the room.

She tried to remember the formula for calculating the centrifugal force. She couldn't. It didn't matter. That was Jessie's cup of tea. Not hers. And suddenly she realized that she, too, was nervous. As nervous as Tom was. Almost but not quite. She got up.

Tom looked at her curiously.

He was curled up into a tight ball in his corner of his own couch. He appeared so vulnerable. His arms were hugging his bent knees.

"What are you doing?" he asked.

"I'm going home," she announced.

He didn't try to talk her out of it.

✳✳✳✳

Her car. A.C.'s car. The 'vette. Where had she parked it?

She remembered. A block away. Dennie walked down the narrow dark street, made even darker and narrower by the construction work with its inevitable wooden fences, scaffolding, and giant yellow machines.

They reminded her of Tonka Toys. Giant Tonka Toys. Why were they supposed to be for boys? She'd loved them. So had her sisters. The real Tonka Toys. They were better than dolls. And these were just like Tonka Toys. Big, overgrown, friendly Tonka Toys.

Except at two in the morning they looked menacing, more like the alien invaders from the "War of the Worlds." They had landed in Chicago this time, not in New Jersey. They had better information. Orson Welles and John Housman had been wrong. No one cared if the martians claimed New Jersey. They could have New Jersey. Newark. Trenton. Paterson. Only William Carlos Williams would mind. And he was dead. That left no one at all.

Dennie reached into her purse and pulled out the car keys.

She heard a noise behind her and tried to duck. Poor reflexes. It was too late. Something smashed into the back of her head.

Something hard.

There was an explosion.

A white light. A floodlight. Flooding her world.

The martians were here.

In full force.

Turning out all the lights in the whole world.

✳✳✳✳

Pain.

Pounding, throbbing pain. Pounding everywhere. Filling her head with noise. Thunder. Endless rolls of thunder.

Starting in the back of her head and then exploding throughout her entire skull. Dennie automatically reached back and touched the source of her agony. Another reflex. One that caused a jolt of pain to burst through her head. Dennie suddenly had new empathy for her sisters and their migraine headaches. Thank God she'd been spared them. Menstrual cramps were enough. Pain. Searing pain. Scorching. Blinding. Pain that enveloped her. Became her. Was her. And then. . . .

✳✳✳✳

She pulled her fingers apart. They felt sticky. They were sticky. She drew her fingers up toward her face. Blood. They were covered with blood. Her blood. Her own blood.

Where was she? She tried to think. She remembered a color. What color? Maize. Maize and blue. No. Not maize. Yellow. Bright yellow. Tonka yellow. She was in Chicago. That much she knew.

But where? Chicago was a big town. A city. With over three million people. Some of whom didn't have pain pounding through their heads. At least a couple of dozen.

The police. She needed the police, but where were they? And where was she? And how could she get from here to there? Or vice versa?

She was on one of the river streets. No, a lake. One of the Great Lakes. Not Michigan. That went north and south. She was going east and west. No, just one way. West. Huron. That was right, Lake Huron. She was on Huron Street. And there were police everywhere. Except where you wanted them to be. And when. There had to be a police station somewhere nearby. There was. At Chicago Avenue. On Chicago Avenue in Chicago, Illinois.

That had to be the closest one. Through the fog and ache that were her brain, Dennie somehow had a distinct image of the precinct on Chicago Avenue. She had never been inside it. She had, in fact, never actually been inside any police station. Beth had. She hadn't. Thank God. This particular one that she had never been inside was on the corner of Chicago and Clark. A couple of blocks west of the Water Tower. There. She knew precisely where it was. She was so proud of herself. How far away that was depended entirely on where she was. That was a much more difficult problem. She tried. Huron. Outside someone's apartment. Whose? Philip Glass. No, it wasn't Philip Glass' apartment. It was somebody else's.

Tom. Tom somebody. On Huron and Dearborn. Huron and Dearborn! That meant that she knew the answer. The Water Tower was only a few blocks away. So was the police station she had to reach. It was the middle of the night. The stores in Water Tower Place wouldn't be open.

Should she walk or drive? She had no idea. Besides, there were more basic questions that had to be addressed first. She knew she was alive. She could feel that much. The hard, rough curb pushing against her face and the damp wet grass was chilling much of the rest of her body. But could she get up? Could she actually walk? Was her car still there? Did she have the keys? Did she have her purse? Her driver's license?

Too many questions. Too complex. They made the pounding worse. She had all she could do to answer one question at a time. There was no need to rush on helter-skelter. The mugger must have gone. Leaving both the scene of the crime and the victim. The scene was doing better than the victim was.

Could she move?

That was the best place to start. Dennie slowly lifted her face off the curb. It felt good to have cool air pushing in on her cheek instead of the rough grain of cement. Without thinking, her left hand came up to rub her left cheek and jaw. The skin was roughened and raw and covered with blood. Her jaw moved freely. Nothing seemed to be broken or out of place. Gingerly, ever so gingerly, she pushed against the ground until she was sitting up.

The world began to rotate in front of her. Left to right. Clockwise. At about two cycles per second. Slow. Steady. Never getting any faster. Or slower. The world rolled by. Trees. Buildings. Streetlights. Tonka trucks. Myriads of the same Tonka truck. The mother of all Tonka trucks.

Dennie felt sick to her stomach. Her body began to sway. Right to left. Counterclockwise. At the same two cycles per second.

Her head dropped forward onto her chest. Her body settled backwards. There was nothing Dennie could do to stop it. She was afraid that she was once again going to crash back into the curb. Into the cement. The rough, hard cement.

She didn't. Instead her body just settled back until she was seated against a smooth surface. Smooth and metallic. The side of a car. What car? Whose car?

She carefully moved her head to get a peek. It was her car. The 'vette. It was still there. It hadn't been stolen. Why not? Maybe the mugger had his own car. Maybe he wasn't into 'vettes. Not like A.C. Or that Eller guy.

Dennie's world stopped spinning in front of her. The cold metal of A.C.'s 'vette pressing against her back felt strangely reassuring. She ought to be able to lift her head.

She tried.

She succeeded.

A sharp jolt of pain shot up from the base of her skull and exploded upward and was gone. One brief flash lasting no more than half an eternity.

Dennie lowered her head until the uninjured side came to rest against the side of the car. The movement didn't precipitate another jolt of pain. It didn't even put the world into motion again. The cold metal felt good against her neck. Her mind was becoming less fog-bound.

The car keys. Where were they? Where were they supposed to be?

In her purse. That's where she always kept them. Her purse! Where was it? She felt the ground. It was next to her. And open. Dennie reached into her purse. There were no keys. No car keys. Not any kind of keys.

Her wallet was there. And her charge cards. And her money. But not the keys. They were gone. But the car was still there.

Why had the mugger taken the car keys and left the car?

Perhaps it wasn't the car keys he was after. It was Dennie's other keys. The keys to her apartment. The keys to Beth's apartment. To their contiguous, racemic apartments.

That was it. The mugger had been after Dennie's other keys. But why? To break into her apartment?

For what?

The back of her head was throbbing. She felt her neck. The goose egg had become a baseball.

The police. The Chicago Avenue police station. She had to get there. And she had to walk there.

Otherwise the mugger might break into her place. And steal something. What? The tapes. That hurt worse than the jolts of lightning that periodically burst out of the base of her skull. She had to prevent that. To do that, she had to get help. To get to the police. Or perhaps to steal something of Beth's. What?

She had no idea.

Dennie staggered to her feet. She knew just where she had to go. West to Clark then straight north to Chicago.

Her world was once again floating by her. It was not a rapid spinning sensation, but more of a gentle turning like one of the bittersweet waltzes of Richard Strauss. No premature explosions. Just an unending series of gentle turns. "Der Rosenkavalier" with tympani and horns.

Dennie could walk. Both legs moved and neither knee gave out. She lurched a bit and staggered but no one was expected to waltz in a straight line. The baseball on her neck was taut and uncomfortable but it was not exploding.

Walking was a cinch. All she had to do was remember to put down the left foot as she lifted the right one and vice versa.

That was easy.

It was almost natural.

And the waltz continued. Slow, swaying.

She lifted her right foot just as her left foot was scheduled to land on the sidewalk. But it didn't. There was no sidewalk. The sidewalk had ended. Her foot had gone beyond the curb. She fell forward as her foot slammed down into the street. The sudden collision snapped her head back and sent a series of painful jolts shooting up from her neck into her head.

The waltz was gone. Replaced by flashes. And throbs. Philip Glass. Driving. Pounding. Exploding.

A volley.

A fusillade.

"The 1812 Overture." Plus "Bolero." At the same time. The entire Second World War. With the original cast. All of them.

Then the world was no longer spinning.

She was.

And there were lights.

Bright lights.

From a car.

Heading toward her.

Closing in on her.

Brakes.

She should be hearing brakes.

She didn't.

All she was aware of were the jolts of pain and the bright lights and the vortex of a spinning world.

Her world.

The end of her world.

And the hard bumper of the car as it crashed into her.

And a name pounding in her head. Philip. Philip Glass.

Chapter
VII

Let me hear the whole story, the voice said. This voice sounded familiar to Dennie. She ought to be able to identify it. Especially now. Afterall, her world was no longer spinning about her and the pounding in her head had subsided into a muffled drum roll and there was no one firing cannons into her neck. Without all those distractions, she surely ought to be able to figure out whose voice it was. But she couldn't. Almost, but not quite. At least she knew where she was; she was flat on her back at the Chicago Avenue police station, staring up at a blank ceiling. And the music had stopped. And at least the ceiling was not made of glass. Just flat white paint. Well, dirty white. Off-white. Far off. No glass. No window. The tapes!

She jerked her head. The world flew by her in a mad whirl. And the pain exploded so loudly she was certain that they heard it in Milwaukee. The voice? Philip Glass. No. There was no Philip Glass. She didn't know any Philip Glass. He wrote music. What was going on in her head was not music. Not "The 1812 Overture." Not "Bolero." Not even Beethoven's Ninth and The Greatful Styx playing simultaneously.

The spinning slowed to a nauseating gyration. Almost a pirouette. Pivoting peacefully. And the pain no longer cried out for morphine. Perhaps nothing stronger than codeine. And someone had shot the drummer. All she could hear was silence. Blessed silence. And above the silence, a voice she ought to be able to place. "Officer Majeski," the voice went on, "I'm waiting."

It was Ward's voice. Tom Ward. Lieutenant Tom Ward. Her friend. Tom. Shy Tom. Tom, who almost requalified as a virgin. Tom Ward was demanding to hear the whole story, like some anxious four-year-old, afraid to miss even a single word. As if magically, the absence of just one word would transform the meaning of all the others or change the ending.

Why was Tom here? He didn't work out of this precinct.

Then Dennie remembered. She had asked them to call Tom Ward. Right before one of the times she'd passed out. They obviously had called him and now he was here. Dennie was tempted to turn her head and look at Tom. She resisted the temptation. There was too much of a chance that any movement on

83

her part would cause a chain reaction of unwanted sensations. It wasn't worth it; she knew what Ward looked like. She just closed her eyes and conjured up his image. Sort of fantasized about him. But with his clothes on.

"Like I told you before, Lieutenant, she just staggered out into the middle of the street," a second voice replied.

That had to be the voice of Officer Majeski. Dennie had no idea at all what Majeski looked like, and she certainly was not interested enough in that question to make any movement whatsoever. And there was no chance at all that she wanted to fantasize about his image. Not with that squeaky tenor voice.

"Yeah," chipped in yet a third male voice. Much deeper. Yet it seemed even younger and more anxious than Majeski's had. "We thought she was some old. . . ," he stopped. She was glad he had. She didn't want to hear the rest. Dennie knew she was recovering. She was as insulted by the "old" as she could possibly have been by the rest, no matter how pejorative.

"I'd turned on the bright lights so she'd notice us," Majeski squeaked on. "I didn't want to use the siren. It was two o'clock. She just kept staggering around. We drove up toward her as slowly as we could and then we stopped the car."

They were certainly not leaving out a single word.

"I was about to get out of the car," the younger, deeper voice broke in. "That's when she spun around like some sort of a whirling dervish and smashed right into our squad car." He might be worth a look. Or a fantasy or two.

"Right into our car," the other voice squeaked.

So that was what had happened. Dennie didn't recall it quite that way. In fact, she hardly had any recall of it at all.

"She didn't seem to be hurt." Majeski's nervousness had turned into an apology. "She'd been mugged. She insisted that we call you. We did. She said you knew her. We didn't believe her about that. She insisted that some guy named Philip Glass had mugged her and left her for dead. It didn't make much sense to us. Her wallet was in her pocket with over two hundred and forty bucks in it. Why would this Glass guy rob her and not take all that dough? Or her credit cards? Unless Glass is some sort of millionaire?"

The voices stopped.

Dennie wanted to hear whatever else they had to say but was glad no one was talking. The silence was soothing. Their words were no longer crashing through her skull and reverberating off her eardrums.

"You two did the right thing. I'm glad you called me." His voice sounded so good to her. "I'm going to talk to Ms. Cater now. If I need your help, I'll call you."

The two policemen sounded relieved, but at the same time disgruntled to be dismissed in such a cavalier fashion. Their feet shuffled as they made their exit.

The door slammed behind them. The loud bang had less ill effect on Dennie than she thought it might. No more than a 5.1 or 5.2 on the Richter scale. No big deal. Hell, she might even try to sit up.

"It wasn't Philip Glass," Dennie said without sitting up. Why push it?

"Philip Glass?"

"The composer. You were playing his songs for me."

"Songs from Liquid Days," he said. "Did you like it?"

"Not that much."

"Start at the beginning," Tom said.

"I was walking to my car," Dennie began. "From your apartment."

"Who knew you were going out with me tonight?"

"You did."

"Anyone else?"

She hadn't told anyone.

"You know what that means?"

She wasn't certain she did.

"Unless this was a random mugging, then someone either knew you'd be there or was trailing you. And no one else knew."

Neither of them believed it was a random mugging. She was getting anxious again. This time she had every right to feel frightened.

"What's missing?"

"My keys." Concentrate.

"Your car keys?" he inquired.

"And the keys to my place," she replied.

"And to Beth's?"

"There's no lock," she reminded him.

"I think we'd better get back to your place. We ought to make sure no one breaks in and takes anything before you get the locks changed. Can you walk?"

She thought she could. "You might have to help me," she added.

"We serve to protect, ma'am."

That was not the right thing to say. Someone had just mugged her. And someone had killed John Doran. Were they the same someone? Did she really need his protection? Would his protection be sufficient? Hell, he didn't even know who to protect her from.

✳✳✳✳

Tom drove Dennie back to her apartment. She hoped that A.C. had another set of keys to the 'vette. If he didn't, she didn't know what she would do. If only Beth were home, she'd know what to do. But she'd better not be. Could she be? Did Dennie have to warn her? No. Beth wouldn't have come home. Beth was too smart to make a mistake like that. Tom Ward parked his car out front in a no parking zone and waited in the car while Dennie went into the security office.

Dennie moved gingerly, being careful not to move her head very much and not to step down very hard. The security guard looked up from his bank of black and white TV screens and actually seemed to recognize her, although she was certain that if she saw him out of context, she would have trouble recognizing him. He was either very unobservant or too polite to comment on the cuts and bruises on her face.

"I've lost my keys," she explained.

"Again," he commented.

"For the first time."

"This week."

"That's my sister."

"You 2A or 2B?"

"2B."

"Too bad. We have lots of spares for 2A. They're in such great demand. Let me check on yours." The guard crossed the hall and went into the office of the building and in a few moments came back to his bank of TV screens dangling a set of keys.

"Good news," he said. "But be careful, we won't be able to get another set made until Monday. So try not to lose these."

"I'll try," she said. "Believe me, I'll try."

✳✳✳✳

As Dennie and Tom approached the door of her apartment, she could see several pieces of paper sticking half way out, under the door.

"Oh, God," she said. "It must be a mess in there. I don't want to see it. Damn. Damn."

Tom said nothing. He hadn't, she realized, since they'd left the police station. Had he suddenly become the strong silent type?

Tom unlocked the door for her. She was afraid to even look in. Tom went inside first. She waited, her back resting against the wall, looking across the hall at Beth's locked door. A couple of pieces of paper were also sticking out from under her door. Beth! Don't be home! Or maybe she'd been home. And. . . .

A moment later Tom called to her from deep inside her apartment. "Nobody's home," he yelled out. His voice sounded good to her. The resonance. And the message. Perhaps he could protect her.

She looked down. The papers were nothing more than a pile of circulars. From competing neighborhood pizza joints. And Chinese restaurants. And her friendly dry cleaners. She bent down and picked them up, trying to ignore the fact that her head was once again spinning. Not as violently as before but still spinning. A pas de deux or two. Nothing too energetic. A slow waltz, perhaps. Johann Strauss. There was no mess at all inside her apartment. Nothing was strewn across the floor. Not so much as a single advertisement. And everything else was also in its place. The books were on the bookshelves. And so were her videotapes. Including the three that were unlabeled. Even the TV was undisturbed. And the CD player. Of course they were. It wasn't some common thief they'd expected. No mugger had grabbed her keys in order to rip off her VCR. The spinning had slowed to a modest wave washing back and forth across her world.

She walked into her bedroom. Her VCR was there. So was her second TV. Despite that, she crossed to her dresser. Her jewelry was there. All of it.

"Everything's okay," she shouted out.

"Everything's okay here, too," Tom called back. He was obviously surveying Beth's apartment. And had obviously not run into Beth. "You sure nothing's missing?" he shouted.

"It looks that way."

When he got back inside her kitchen, he picked up the phone there and punched in a number. "A locksmith," he explained. "We use him all the time. I'll tell him to install a new dead bolt lock for you."

She maneuvered her way back into the living room. The waves were getting deeper now. So were the troughs. Like tidal waves. Or were those the crests? And pounding had also built up. It had become a crescendo. Like some Philip Glass version of the "Anvil Chorus." And the pain. It, too, was pounding. To a different rhythm. She fell into the couch.

"Dennie," Tom's voice startled her. "Go to bed."

"What? Oh." She struggled to get up. The waves were going around in circles. Like a whirlpool. No, a whirligig. Only counterclockwise. Like the water in a toilet below the equator. But who had flushed it? With her head in it? Tom was supposed to protect her. To save her. She needed saving. Now!

"Bed. The locksmith will be here at one. I'll call you at twelve thirty."

She was standing. She could stand up. No mean feat, that. She could stand up by herself. On her own two feet. But why was Tom swaying in circles. Around and around. Like a maelstrom. What a good word. Like the vortex of a maelstrom. No, more like a carousel. Or as if he were on a ferris wheel. Going faster and faster. He was twirling. And swaying. And falling. He was going to fall. He grabbed her by the arm. He'd be safe now. She'd keep him from falling.

Hold on tight!

He held on tight.

Now they were both swaying. Round and round. Faster and faster. Like two tops. Or one top. Or a whirling dervish. Or two dervishes. Rotating dervishes. Performing a dance. Some sort of circle dance. A gyration. Going faster and faster. In a small circle. An ever-narrowing gyre.

Like witches. Witches dancing. Witches dancing around a fire. A bonfire. And howling. Howling. And spinning faster and faster. Building up to something. To a climax.

Tom was no longer holding her up. He was pushing her down. Down. Down onto something soft. Onto a bed. She was no longer spinning.

She was lying down now. Or was she laying down? Did it matter? She was on her back. On a bed. Flat on her back on a bed. The rest of the word was spinning around her.

Above her was a figure. A man. A big man. This big man. Who? Who this time? Tom. He was above her. His face was all that she could see. A face coming down on her. Bearing down on her. A whirling face. It was all she could see. But not all she could feel. He was pulling her clothes off. First her shoes. She didn't need them anyway.

Then her skirt. Why was he doing that? Why? Why that way? Why so roughly? And why didn't he stop? Pulling. Yanking. Her skirt.

Her jacket. And why was he still staring down at her?

Then her blouse. Button by button. It was open. It was gone. Pulled away from her. She was now frozen in place. Afraid to move. Afraid to even speak. Now he was doing something else. To her legs. Pulling them apart. Far apart. Together. She had to keep them together. She willed them to stay together. Her knees. Her thighs. They wouldn't. They didn't. Apart. Open. Splayed open.

And everything was throbbing. Her head. Her neck. Her chest. All of her. And spinning. The whole world was in the vortex that was her maelstrom.

She tried to say something. To stop him. To stop the spinning. To scream. She wanted to open her mouth and scream. Nothing came out. If she opened it, then. . . .

He was now over her. Pulling something toward her face. Toward her mouth. Closed. She had to keep it closed. Pressure. Her throat. Nausea. Gagging. No. NO. NO!

She passed out.

✳✳✳✳

Bells. Bells. The tintinnabulation of the bells. But they weren't bells. And they weren't tintinnabulating. They were rings and they were pealing more than ringing. Celebrating a victory. Whose? Over whom? Or were they tolling? For whom? She was afraid to ask. She knew the answer all too well. She had always known that answer. Tolling. Reverberating inside her skull. An entire carillon. A cathedral full of bells. One bell. Not even a real bell. A phone. Her own phone. And it was ringing for her.

And she was in her own bed. Undressed. And all tucked in.

She picked up the phone.

"You okay?" the voice asked. It was Tom Ward's voice. Identified in an instant this time.

"Yes," she said, guessing that she was. At least she did know that she was in her own bed. "Why?"

"Your phone has been ringing for five minutes," he replied. "I was getting worried."

"That's nice."

"The locksmith will be there in less than half an hour."

The locksmith. What locksmith? Then she remembered. The mugging. The police station. Tom. The keys. The spinning. The bed. Tom! Above her. Pulling at her clothes. Coming toward her. Yanking at her legs. . . . She tore off the quilt that was pulled up to her chin.

She had on her bra. And her panties. She obviously had not undressed herself. She would not have left those on. Who had? She remembered, shivering as she did. Tom. Tom had.

"Tom. Did you. . . ?"

"Did I . . . what?" he asked rather coldly.

"I mean did . . . did we. . . ?"

"Did we what?"

They obviously hadn't. Why not? Hadn't he found her attractive enough? Maybe if she exercised as much as Beth.

"We still have a deal, don't we?" he asked.

"A deal?"

"You were going to leave the Krollers to me."

The Krollers? She tried to dredge up the name and the deal. The Krollers. That cold man and his cold wife. It all came back to her. She pulled her quilt up to her chin. It didn't help.

"I deal with Leslie and that Havergal somebody."

"Big Brian Havergal."

"That's the one," she said proudly. She was very much back on track.

"Be careful."

"I'm too old for him."

"Dennie!"

Tom's warning was probably justified but it was not exactly what she had wanted to hear at that moment.

✳✳✳✳

At exactly one-o-one, Dennie let the locksmith in. He hardly gave her a first look and certainly not a second one. She was glad. Her face looked ghastly. Scraped. Swollen. Bloody. No wonder Tom had not wanted to take off all of her clothing. Her face would stop romance. Cold. And probably lust, too. She returned to her bathroom and washed her face again. Gently but thoroughly. Then she covered up as much of the damage as she could with makeup. Face powder. Base. Whatever she had. Only when she was done did she dare to look at herself again. Not quite so bad. Not bad at all. She had the Michael Jackson look. Only she was several shades darker. And she wore less lipstick. But it worked.

While the locksmith was still locksmithing away, doing whatever it was that locksmiths do, she replayed the tape of Leslie's last session with John Doran. It was the list she wanted. The list of witches. They, too, could all be considered to be suspects. They had all been participants in the witchcraft rituals. That made them accessories. Accessories to rape. The rape of Leslie English. And who knows to how many others. And to what else.

It took only a few minutes to find the right place on the tape where Leslie had told the names to John Doran. She listened and wrote out the names. One by one.

Collins. Risberg. Weaver. Felsch. Gandil. McMillan. Lynn. Williams. Russell. Danforth. Scott. Berger.

She listened to the tape again. And rechecked her list. She had gotten the names right. She was done. And so was the locksmith. He gave her three keys, but no bill.

"What do I owe you?" she asked him.

"Your life."

"My life?"

"A private joke," he said.

"Then why aren't I laughing?"

"Sorry. I thought you knew. I'm a police officer. I usually padlock crime sites. Ward told me this was official business."

Official business. Did that mean that she'd be safe from everyone who wasn't on official police business? Everyone but Tom Ward. And the rest of the cops. Tom Ward, she didn't mind. Not that he seemed all that interested. "Is padlocking the scene of a crime pretty standard?"

"Depends on the crime."

"Murder."

"And the location?" the locksmith added noncommittally.

"In an office space? One that wouldn't be used?"

"Pretty common," he told her.

"SOP?" she persisted.

"Not SOP, but if the office would be closed, or if it's in a quiet place, then it's pretty much SOP," he concluded.

SOP. But not in this case. Why not? A single possibility occurred to Dennie. One that must have been on the edge of her consciousness. Had she been set up? To take one tape. But she had taken four. Tom only knew about one. How could that be?

The other tapes!

The locksmith said goodbye and closed the door behind him. Locking it.

Locking it! He had a key! Some security. What should she do next? Leslie. She called Leslie. She was home, but preoccupied.

"What am I going to do now?" Leslie pleaded. "Without Mr. Doran."

"We'll just have to find another expert witness. He didn't want to testify anyway."

"That's not what I meant. You sound just like Sean Keneally. That's what he said. He'd find me some other expert. I'm not interested in an expert. I'm not worried about that damn lawsuit now. I'm worried about me. Me! He's dead. He was my therapist. He helped me. He understood me. I need him! Where am I going to find another therapist like that?" She was crying now. Hard. Dennie could feel her emotion. It seemed real. But she'd been fooled by tears before.

"Help me. Please." The young woman's pleas sounded more like those of a hurt little girl. A frightened little girl. About to panic.

"I will," Dennie promised her. "I'll help you find someone."

"Thank you," she sniffed, sounding reassured. "Did you want something?"

She'd almost forgotten. "The list."

"What list?"

Dennie hated doing this. Especially now, but it had to be done. "The list of names. The names you told Mr. Doran. Do you remember?"

"The witches," she said bitterly.

"Yes, the list of witches. Those twelve names."

"Plus my mother. She was the thirteenth. And thirteen made it a coven. That was what Mr. Doran explained to me." Leslie was once again sobbing audibly.

"Do the names mean anything to you?"

"I don't know. I can't remember them all."

Dennie hesitated. She took a deep breath. She'd try another tactic. There was no need to be nondirective. This was not therapy and she wasn't Leslie's therapist.

"Let me read you the list. You tell me which ones you recognize."

"Okay."

Dennie started. "Collins," she said, and then she waited.

Leslie said nothing.

"Risberg," followed by another pause. "Weaver."

"We had some neighbors by that name. The Weavers. They lived across the street from us."

"When?"

"When I was a little girl."

That information did not surprise Dennie. That was the right time period. "Felsch."

"Felsch?"

"Yes."

"She was my best friend in first grade. Or kindergarten. One of them. I can just barely remember her. We were just little kids. She was always smiling. We all called her Happy. That was her nickname. Happy Felsch."

"What was her real name?"

"Robbie . . . no, Roberta, I think."

"What happened to her?"

"They moved away. And. And. Oh, God. I do know what happened to her. She killed herself. In high school. Oh, my God."

Roberta had not been that happy. But Leslie had known her. That meant two so far. Two out of four. And both from early childhood. Back to the list. "Gandil."

No response. They were down to two out of five.

"McMillan."

"That brat. We went to grammar school together. He was a brat. Still is, I bet."

The same grammar school. That meant they'd lived in the same neighborhood. Quite a coincidence. Hell, it was not a coincidence at all. Where had she thought the witches came from? Had they all flown in for the rituals? On their broomsticks? Of course not. They were friends. Neighbors. Those block parties must have really been something. Block parties from hell.

"Lynn." That name meant nothing to her.

"Williams." More neighbors. They had two girls. Twins. Four or five years older. One was now in medical school at Austin Flint. They had been her babysitters for a while.

"Russell."

She did not remember that name.

"Danforth."

"Gerri! She was my best friend."

"I thought Happy was?"

"She was."

Dennie understood. They were all best friends.

"Berger."

"No."

They were done. Leslie made her repeat her promise to help her find a therapist. Dennie said she would. They said goodbye. How would she find a therapist for her?

She next called Paul Richardson. He was in with a patient but he took her call. She identified herself. And he remembered her. She wanted to talk to him about witchcraft.

Would tomorrow morning be okay? About nine?

Nine was okay with her. Where?

His office. At Austin Flint.

Dennie looked at the list. At the coven. Leslie had recognized five of the names. Weaver, the neighbor. And not so Happy Felsch. Her best friend. As a little girl. Brat McMillan. The Williams twins. And her one-time best friend, Gerri Danforth. According to Leslie, one of the Williams twins was a medical student at Austin Flint. Austin Flint! Dennie bet they had a page operator at Austin Flint.

When Kim Williams answered her page, Dennie lied to her. It was a good way to start up a relationship. She was a friend of Leslie's. She was interested in applying to medical school. Leslie remembered that Kim was at Austin Flint and suggested they might get together and talk and she was going to be at Austin Flint tomorrow.

In no time it was arranged. They'd meet for breakfast at seven thirty.

"How is Leslie?"

"She's okay."

"I haven't seen her for years. Funny. She and my younger sister were friends. I used to babysit for her."

Her younger sister. Leslie had only mentioned the twins. Not the other sister. Why? Playing detective was so much fun, she thought, as she hung up the phone. Except you got beat up sometimes.

She had one more call to make. She had to call A.C. downstairs in the garage. A.C. was there. Didn't she love that 'vette?

She did. Did he have an extra set of keys? He did. But why did she need them? She'd left hers at some guy's apartment and, well. . . . Enough said. Anytime.

She put labels on the three unlabeled tapes and took the one she had already seen and one other and put them into a laundry bag. The third she labeled "Family Vacation—Salem" and put it back on the shelf. She put on her leather jacket. She looked outside. It was raining. A cold February rain. A cold windy February rain. The kind that chilled her to the marrow. As if her marrow were not already suffering from frostbite.

She dropped off the tapes at her dry cleaner. And picked up the keys from A.C. She'd bring the car back within the hour.

"No problem," A.C. said. "The meter's running."

That was the problem.

Now all she had to do was get a cab. Easier said than done on a cold, rainy, windy day in February. In the Windy City. She stood in the doorway. A man joined her. He looked familiar, sort of. She'd seen him before. Very familiar. Those eyes. But not the lips. He had to be a neighbor. One of the myriad of yuppies. In all probability some sort of lawyer. Or a trader. No, he seemed too nice for that.

They waited together.

"The hotel," he said. "Across the street and down the block. The doorman there will get us cabs."

That sounded like a good idea to her.

Neither of them had an umbrella and the rain gave no signs of letting up. And an umbrella wouldn't have helped in that wind. "Let's get out of here," he insisted.

"It's still raining," Dennie complained. "My hair will get frizzy." To say nothing of what it would do to her makeup. What did Michael Jackson do in the rain?

"But it doesn't look like it's going to stop," he replied.

He pushed his way through the revolving door. Dennie followed him. They walked quickly. The hotel was in the middle of the next block. If they walked quickly they would only get slightly soaked instead of totally drenched. The rain didn't seem to bother him. It bothered her. It was making a mess of her makeup. And the wind was cutting right through her.

The light at the corner was red.

"I knew it'd be red," Dennie said. "They're always red when it rains and I'm not wearing a rain coat or a rain hat or carrying an umbrella. It's always that way." Each drop that fell on her seemed to increase her anger.

The lawyer did not agree with her. Traffic lights were red at least half the time, he pointed out. No matter what the weather was. It was not an act of a malevolent god nor some conspiracy. At least not one he understood.

Nor was the rain.

Maybe he was a trader.

Things like that just happened to people. More often than not.

He was probably right. She tried to pretend that the rain felt good. That the small drops that struck her face were refreshing, and in a way they were. She felt more awake than she had before, more alive than she had in days. Her senses were being stimulated. It felt good to be able to feel the cold rain. Good to be alive. Better than the alternative. Far better. She would call Tom. And Beth. She'd try to get in touch with Beth.

The rain washed over her like a fine mist.

Splat.

That was not mist.

Nor rain.

Dennie felt something hit her shoulder. That lawyer was wrong. They were mere victims waiting for whatever God sent down upon them. And now the rain had been replaced by hailstones. Nothing else hit that hard.

She waited to hear the rattle of falling ice against the sidewalk, the ping of hail against the manhole covers. Could that, too, be called tintinnabulation? She listened. She heard nothing.

Splat.

She'd been hit again. On her right shoulder this time. She jerked her head automatically. Not that she expected to see anything. Hail just bounced off and bounced away.

It had not been a hailstone. There was something on the shoulder of her black leather jacket. A glob of gray-white granular gunk.

She felt it. It was cement. Fresh cement. Fresh wet cement. On her leather jacket.

The cement had descended from the new office building that was being built to obstruct her view of the Chicago skyline. Such as it was. She looked up toward the building. It was a skeleton of steel beams coated with cement and half hidden in the low hanging clouds.

Swat.

More cement.

On her skirt this time. Her favorite black skirt. Her dry cleaner was going to get more business than they had expected. The red light seemed to last forever. The lawyer had put his hand on her shoulder.

"My name is Cater," she said. "Dennie Cater."

He said nothing in reply. She felt another splat.

"You bastard," she shouted up at her anonymous assailant and looked up into the fog over them.

Something was careening toward her.

Directly toward her.

Her and the lawyer.

It was not cement this time.

It was the whole damn steel cement bucket.

Cascading right down on her. Careening toward her. Toward them. The hand tightened around her shoulder.

"Look out," the lawyer shouted.

The light changed.

He shoved her.

A Toyota started moving.

Its brakes screeched.

She bounced into its bumper and slid to the pavement. The lawyer jumped backwards and hit the building.

The cement bucket crashed into the sidewalk just where she had been standing. And a crack appeared in the sidewalk. About the size of the San Andreas Fault.

"Christ!" she said, staggering to her feet, as a shower of cement flew in every direction. Dennie watched in silent awe as the crack spread. That could have been her head. Or his. She wasn't hurt. She swallowed hard. The lawyer also looked as if he had not been hurt. His coat had been torn. Big deal.

She was standing up. She was wetter than ever now and covered with cement, but she was unscathed. "I'm okay, I think. How about you?"

"What the fuck?" he replied eloquently. "The wind. It must have blown that bucket down."

That had to be what had happened. "I'm soaked," she said.

"The wind," he reiterated. He was still shaking. It had just missed them. The heavy steel bucket had shattered the sidewalk. It would have killed both of them. Her heart was pounding. And her head. And the spinning was beginning again.

"Are you sure you're okay?" he asked her.

"Yes," she said, not completely confident that she was.

They were both standing there next to the curb, getting wetter. But at least no more cement was falling.

"The wind," he said, shaking his head.

"That weren't no wind. No way, man," a third voice said.

The voice surprised them both. They had considered this to be their own private nightmare. The voice belonged to a black kid, no more than fourteen or fifteen years old, wearing cut-off blue jeans, a red Chicago Bulls T-shirt with number 23 on it, and Nike shoes. Air Jordans, of course. The T-shirt and jeans were covered with splotches of gray cement. But not the Air Jordans. They had a few telltale streaks to show where the cement had been before it had been removed.

"No wind, man," the kid repeated. "A dude. A cool dude. Cooler than you. And a lot blacker."

A cool dude!

Had there been an accident of some sort?

"A real cool dude. Skinheaded. He done pushed that bucket."

Dennie was certain he must have been one of the workmen. He must have slipped.

"He done kicked the bucket. And so did you."

Dennie looked at the kid. His eyes were glazed. His pupils were constricted. He was spaced out on some form of dope. Even on a clear day he'd have trouble seeing the top of the building. And the day was not clear. The top of the building was shrouded in mist and clouds. And the kid was totally out of it. He couldn't possibly know what he saw. Or could he?

The light changed again. The kid walked away, dribbling an imaginary ball, first with his right hand, then his left, then between his legs.

"Are you sure he kicked it?" she yelled after him.

"A cool dude dood it."

"That's why it's called the Windy City," the lawyer concluded, trying to make light of their near mishap.

She started to tell him that the nickname had nothing to do with the weather, but he was halfway across the street.

And she was still shaking so much she couldn't move.

Chapter
VIII

Dennie wanted to go home, to get undressed, to crawl into her own bed and just lie there all by herself. Forever. Or at least until it all went away. And it was Spring. A permanent Spring. It wasn't going to go away. Even if Spring came early. That wasn't what a real detective would do. Not Sam Spade. He wouldn't give it all up and call it a day just because some dude had tried to kill him by pushing a steel cement bucket off a roof. That was nothing more than a minor inconvenience. His day would be just starting. Well, this might be his cup of tea, but it wasn't hers. The indefatigable SOB. Nor would Spencer. Dudes and goons tried to knock him off in every book. Spencer at least had a steady girlfriend. Or at least he did in the earlier books. The ones she liked better. He also had the Hawk to protect him. What did she have? Too damn little. One sister recovering from a nervous breakdown. One sister scared and running. Well, she was scared, too. Why couldn't she run and hide?

She was a woman. All alone. Alone in Chicago. V.I. Warshawski. She would not give up so easily. Chicago's own. It was funny that she had the same name as an auto supply company. Auto parts. Mufflers. Tires. Transmissions. That sort of thing. Warshawski. Perhaps they were related. Nor would Mike Hammer. But they were all real detectives. Dennie wasn't a detective. She had no license. No credentials at all. No experience. She didn't even own a gun. Guns scared her. Nothing Freudian there. It was real guns she disliked. And she sure as hell wasn't hard-boiled. Beth was the one with the hard shell.

Was Beth safe? If some dude wanted to kill her, that same goon probably wanted to kill Beth. Why? For the same reason. Whatever that was. Except more so. Beth might know something. Really know something.

Beth hadn't called her. Dennie felt even more chilled than before. And more frightened. For both of them. Was Beth even still alive? Dennie hadn't heard from her since the murder. Except for that tape. And the fax to Sean. Where was she? Alone? Tired? Frightened? Or . . . or with Mike? She had to call Mike. But not from her bugged phone.

That drugstore across the street had to have a phone. She crossed the street. It did. And she had plenty of quarters.

Mike would be at work. She dialed Mike's work number.

"Sergeant O'Rourke," the voice answered.

"Mike."

"None other. And to whom do I have the pleasure of speaking?"

"Dennie," she said. "Dennie Cater."

"I knew which Dennie it was," Mike rasped, and then coughed once.

"You should stop smoking."

"You sound just like your darling sister."

"That's why I called. About Beth."

"Did you hear from her?" Mike asked anxiously.

"No. Did you?"

"Of course," Mike coughed out and then paused.

"Mike, how is she?"

"Fine," Mike said, suddenly sounding very, very official. "All in order, Ms."

"You can't talk?" she asked.

"That's right."

"Did you see her?"

"No, I didn't, Ms." Very, very official now.

"She's not at your place?"

"No, not yet."

Not yet! "But she called? And she will be?"

"That's correct."

"And she's okay. And she's going to see you. Thank God."

"Excuse me."

All she heard was some muffled mumbling. But she knew that Beth was safe. And was going to see Mike. When? What difference did that make?

"I must go now," Mike said. "Lieutenant Ward is here."

Ward! Why? What did Ward know about Mike? How? Did it matter? Dennie had learned what she'd wanted to learn. Beth was okay. Beth was safe. It was time to go home and crawl into bed, by herself. At least until she stopped shaking.

✳✳✳✳

The answering machine was flashing. Dennie pushed PLAY. It rewound itself and there was Beth. Beth! "Hi, kid. I'm fine. I'm safe. But you be careful. I saw it all. Someone pushed that cement bucket. It was no accident. That dopehead was right."

Someone! Who? Beth had seen it all. She must have been right there. And she had just missed her. Damn!

"A black guy," Beth continued. "Over six feet. Very muscular. A big guy. Looked like a linebacker. Real tough type. With his scalp all shaved."

Like Horace Eller.

"He looked sort of like Horace Eller."

How did Beth know what Horace Eller looked like? Beth was the detective in the family And she was trying to dig up anything and everything that might help Leslie. Anything about Doran. Or the Krollers. Kroller! The daughter rapist! The same Kroller who employed goons like Horace. And not to play linebacker. But to terrorize people. Well, she was sure as hell terrorized. How had she ever thought she liked him?

"Be careful, kid. You're the one who holds us all together. I'd die if anything happened to you."

So would I if. . . .

"I know how to take care of myself. And so does Mike. Mike takes care of me better than anyone else ever did. Except you. But this is so different. God, I'm getting sentimental. Me, getting sentimental. I'm beginning to sound like you. Or Jessie. Whew. That's scary. That must be because I'm scared."

Beth—scared?

"I'm frightened for you. Take care of yourself I'm going to try to keep an eye on you as much as I can. You're so damn naive. So trusting. In this world you can't trust anybody. By the way, I talked to Mike. We're going to get together. But I can't say anything more. Mike says that our phone may be bugged."

"Sayonara, as James Michener would have said. Sayonara, kid. Take care."

CLICK.

BEEP. BEEP. BEEP.

That was her only message.

Beth was safe. That was all that really mattered. Dennie didn't need any other messages. And Beth was looking after her. Not exactly the Hawk, but it was a start. She wasn't as alone as she thought.

But she had more reason to be frightened. The falling bucket hadn't been an accident. No more than the mugging had been random. She had been mugged for a reason. The mugger had specifically mugged her. And now someone had almost killed her. Thank God for that lawyer who pushed her. He saved her life. He never even introduced himself. A twentieth century Lone Ranger. Ward. Tom Ward. She had to tell him.

Or did she?

Not if her phone was bugged. Tom would already know. If not now, pretty soon. Perhaps she wouldn't tell him and see what developed. Pretty clever girl.

Beth would be proud of her. So would Jessie. God, she couldn't wait until the three of them could all be together again. Like the three Musketeers.

All for one. One for all. Plus D'Artagnan. Who was their D'Artagnan? Mike? No, not Mike. Mike was no Erroll Flynn.

Tom? He had possibilities. Tom, whom she wasn't going to tell about the cement bucket? Or the big black goon who had tried to kill her? Dennie was shivering again. And she was very scared. She needed more protection than a fugitive Beth might be able to provide her.

And she was also wet. And in pain. Her face hurt. And her neck. And the back of her head. And the spinning was once again there in the background and trying to make that background into foreground.

And she was alone.

All alone. Too goddamn alone. Thank God Beth was alright. And thank all the gods and all the saints that Jessie wasn't even involved in this mess. Poor delicate vulnerable Jessie. Safe in Wisconsin. She missed Jessie. And Beth. She couldn't even talk to them. And she had no idea what the hell she should do. Except take off her clothes, crawl into bed, and have a good cry.

V.I. wouldn't do that.

To hell with her. She wasn't V.I. She was Dennie Cater. And sometimes a good cry helped. She pulled down the quilt and started taking off her clothes. And the tears started flowing. Washing away her makeup. Her Michael Jackson look. Michael Jackson with tears.

✳✳✳✳

The library at DePaul was not exactly the Library of Congress. Nor the library of the British Museum. So what? She wasn't exactly Karl Marx. And she certainly wasn't trying to write *Das Kapital.* She just wanted to do a little research on witchcraft. And Brian Havergal. And this was the only place that combined both. Or at least the possibility of both.

It was time to start her quest. Her game. The game. The game she hated so. No wonder Beth refused to play the game. Luckily she'd found Mike so she no longer had to. Dennie took off her long woolen winter coat. The one she'd worn as an undergraduate. She plucked it out from the back of her closet as part of her disguise as a student. A poor but sexy student. God, she hated this game. She hated wearing a skirt that was too tight and too short. And black panty hose. All just to attract men. Thank God she had good legs. And didn't have to wear a sweater that was too tight or a neckline that went down to her navel or both.

She picked out a table near the entrance. She put her coat on one chair. Along with her book bag. Another remnant from college. Then she angled that chair toward her and away from the table, pulled a couple of books from the book bag, sat down and stretched out, her legs coming to rest on the book bag.

Stretched to their fullest. In full view of the door. God, she felt like that character from "The Graduate." Mrs. Robinson revisited. She'd watched that movie so many times with her dad. He loved it. She'd learned to like it. And now she was Mrs. Robinson. Only younger and not quite as thin. And with panty hose. Not nylons.

She had to start reading. She grabbed a book. Sylvia Plath. She'd never liked Sylvia Plath. It was Beth's old book bag. Beth, she reminded herself, was fine! Had that been Beth following her during the cab ride to the 'vette? And then the short trip here and the eternal search for a parking space? It had to have been. She was not entirely alone.

On to Sylvia Plath.

"Hi," he said. He was young. Too young. Not much more than barely out of his teens. If that. Far too young for her.

"I'm George Etten. I'm a sophomore here," he said with a smile.

Absolutely too young. Twenty tops.

"I'm sure I've seen you around campus."

"Denise," she said, not too smartly. "Denise . . . Eller." Why that name?

"I'm pre-law," he said.

"I'm not." None too brightly. She really was not good at this. "I'm a psych major." Not a complete lie. "But only part-time. I work as a paralegal."

"Must be interesting."

He wasn't much better at it.

"We must have had a class together. What psych courses did you take last quarter? I took one."

"None. I just started."

"Oh." He actually sounded disappointed.

Did he really believe that he'd seen her around campus? One pair of long legs with black panty hose stretched out on a chair was pretty much like any other. And with all that makeup on even her own mother would have trouble recognizing her. And all he was looking at were her thighs. "Maybe it was at a basketball game," she suggested.

"Maybe," he answered, without much enthusiasm.

"I just love watching Brian play."

"You and the rest of the girls. Mind if I sit down?"

She started to shift her legs.

"No, I'll sit here," he said, pulling out the next chair. No reason to ruin his view.

They talked for twenty minutes. In that twenty minutes she found out quite a lot. Brian was a real lady's man. He was famous for one-night stands. He was apparently working his way through the entire female student body.

"Not us part-time students," she half complained.

"He'll get to you, don't worry. Or maybe you should worry."

"Why?"

"Nothing. Just jealousy, I guess."

"I'm not into one-nighters," she said very truthfully.

"Me neither. But he is. In a big way. And from what I've heard, he doesn't take no for an answer."

He didn't want to say anymore.

She let it drop.

He then got what he wanted. Her phone number. And she got what she wanted. His code numbers for the library's computers. And his library computer card. She'd misplaced hers.

Wouldn't he need it?

No. The librarians all knew him. Besides he'd get it back when they went out for coffee.

She agreed. What choice did she have? He was not as naive as she had thought. And he didn't believe in one-night stands. But he was so damn young. Not young enough to play Dustin Hoffman to her Mrs. Robinson. But still too young.

She went over to one of the self-help computers. And with a little self-help from one of the librarians, she got just what she wanted. A computerized search of the entire medical literature for witchcraft. A Medline search, it was called. And it contained all entries from 1966 through 1993. There were a total of fifty-four entries. If she had a billing number, it would print them all out for her. All fifty-four of them.

She did. So she typed it in. And it typed them out in only a couple of minutes. She took the long strip of computer paper and sat down at a different desk. One occupied by two women who looked to be her age. Grad students, not sophomores.

She started with the first reference. The article was written by somebody named Schoeneman. "Criticisms of the psycho-pathological interpretation of witch hunts: a review." It had been published in the *American Journal of Psychiatry* in 1982. A review article was always a good place to start. There was even an abstract of the article in the printout. Dennie read it, but there was far too much jargon for her. What did it mean? That we used to believe that the mentally ill were witches? So what? That wasn't what she was after. Not at all.

She was after witches. Witches as a cause. Not a result. Not witchcraft as an interpretation. But witchcraft causing mental illness. Depression. Schizophrenia. Neuroses. Whatever. Especially depression. And dreams. Nightmares.

She scanned the list. She found one that seemed to be what she wanted. It was by an author named Weiner. The title seemed good. "The influence of others: witchcraft as an explanation of behavioral disturbances." Witchcraft as a cause, not as an interpretation. That was what she was after. It was in something called *J Nerv Ment Dis* from 1973. *Journal of Nervous and Mental Disease.* She put an asterisk next to the listing. There was no abstract in the printout. There was nothing for her to read. She had to go by the title alone. She needed that article. Where could she get it? She went up to the librarian and asked. This was not a medical library, she was told. They'd have to request it. And that might take a couple of weeks.

Did any libraries in Chicago have that journal?

The librarian checked her computer. The University of Chicago, the University of Illinois, and Austin Flint.

Dennie knew where she'd go. She went back to the table and continued down the printout. She found another interesting title. "Dysesthesia, witchcraft, and conversion reaction. A case successfully treated with psychotherapy." Witchcraft as cause again. Witchcraft that had been treated. Shades of the late John Doran. It was written by two authors named Hilliard and Rockwell. It had been published in the *Journal of the American Medical Association.* In 1978.

Dennie systematically worked her way through all fifty-four entries. There were only three that seemed to have to do with witchcraft as a cause of psychiatric disease. That surprised her. It was such a very short list. There was the one by Weiner in the *Journal of Nervous and Mental Disease* from 1973, "Witchcraft as a cause of behavioral disturbances." Then the one by Hilliard and Rockwell in *JAMA* in 1978. "Witchcraft as a cause of dysesthesia." The best one was by a Heinrich Weber from the *Journal of Cultural Analysis* in 1990. "Witchcraft as a cause of multiple personality disorder." Once again no abstract. But that one sounded the most promising.

That was it. Not exactly a preponderance of data. Maybe Richardson knew of more articles. More data. He'd written an article about witchcraft. Tom had told her that. That was why she was going to talk to him. She didn't remember coming across it on her printout. She rechecked it. The Medline search had missed that one.

Why? She'd have to ask Paul Richardson.

But now it was time to get back to another question. Big Brian Havergal. The man who wouldn't take no for an answer. Dennie struck up a conversation with the two women at her table. Did either of them know Brian Havergal?

One did. The one with the lighter sweater. And bigger breasts.

That figured.

They'd gone out on one date.

Was he as . . . as . . . as big?

Bigger. And better.

So much for feminism.

But.

But what?

"He doesn't take no for an answer," the other girl interrupted.

"Who wants to say no?" the first girl asked.

"Does he get violent?" Dennie asked.

"He doesn't have to," she cooed.

So much for equal rights.

✳✳✳✳

Dennie's answering machine was again winking at her. She had two messages. The first was from Tom Ward. He wanted her to call him at home after
seven. And he had left his home number. The second was from George Etten.
He, too, wanted her to call him at home after seven. He was cute. And it was
after seven. She called Tom Ward.

"I've been trying to call you all day," he opened.

Funny, she got only one message.

"You okay?" he continued.

Yes, why was he asking?

"That was quite a blow on the head you got."

"I'm fine," she said, half unconsciously touching the egg at the base of her
skull. It was getting smaller. And less tender. Not that less tender, she winced.
She also rotated her head once moderately slowly. The room made only two
gyrations. And she didn't even want to retch. She was better.

"Our deal," he said, changing the subject.

Deal? "I haven't done much. I talked to Leslie about those names."

"Names?"

"The names of the twelve witches. She remembered some of them." She
then brought him up to date. She'd tell him more when she knew something
more substantive. She also told him what she'd learned about Brian
Havergal.

"Stay away from him," he said.

"Is that professional advice? Or personal?"

He ignored her question.

Had he learned anything?

Perhaps. He had a tape to show her. From Doran's office. Someone had used the keys to the office to get inside. Those had probably been her keys. The ones she'd used. The mugging may have been to get those keys. The keys to Doran's office. Not her keys.

She made no reply.

He'd show her his tape if she showed him hers.

"Which tape?" she asked.

"You know," he informed her.

She wished she did. When?

Tonight.

She was too tired.

He was persistent. Tomorrow, she suggested. Around noon.

Where? "Your place or mine?"

"Mine," she said. She'd been to his place once and, considering what she had gotten out of it, a return visit didn't seem too inviting.

"I'll bring lunch," he said. "And be careful. I don't want anybody to hit you with another cement bucket."

He knew about the cement bucket. Her phone was bugged. That's how he knew about the cement bucket. And Beth. And Mike. MIKE!

Thank God she'd called Mike from a pay phone. Beth had used Mike's name. But there were a lot of Mikes in Chicago.

"Noon," she said.

"Both," he said.

"Both what?"

"Both professionally and personally."

✳✳✳✳

When Mike opened the door, Beth was there. Waiting.

"My darling girl," Mike said.

"I love you," Beth said.

"And I, you."

"Hug me."

They hugged.

"Kiss me."

They kissed.

"Make love to me."

"I will and you will make love to me."

That sounded like a perfect arrangement to both of them.

Chapter
IX

No one was waiting for her at the entrance to the 800 Club at Austin Flint Medical Center. She asked the receptionist for Ms. Kim Williams.

"Dr. Kim Williams," she was told, and then the receptionist pointed to a young woman seated alone at a table for two that was along the window. Behind her was a spectacular view of the Chicago skyline and a dull orangish-yellow sun beginning to peak through from behind the clouds and mist of a gray winter morning. When would the season change for the better?

Kim Williams was wearing a short white coat. That, Dennie assumed, was what marked her as a medical student even if the receptionist had referred to her as a doctor. Dr. Kim Williams was short and thin. With short, sandy hair. And tired eyes. Very tired. As if she had not slept in several nights. She was probably about Dennie's age. Did Dennie look that tired? She hoped not.

Kim Williams didn't look up until Dennie had sat down opposite her. "Hi," she said flatly.

Not exactly the red carpet treatment. "Hi," Dennie responded, not too cheerfully. Some days were better left somber. "I'm Dennie Cater." With that she extended her hand.

Kim shook hands reluctantly, hesitantly, unenthusiastically. Limply. Disinterestedly. Or was she just plain exhausted? Sometimes people were just tired. Especially medical students.

"Sorry I'm late," Dennie went on.

Kim said nothing. She was looking at her half-empty coffee cup, ignoring the sun that was beginning to burn its way through to the skyline and the life beyond it.

The waitress came by and refilled Kim's coffee cup, poured coffee for Dennie, and took their orders. Orange juice and oatmeal.

The interruption didn't change much. Kim was now staring at a full cup of coffee. In almost no time at all the two glasses of orange juice arrived. And with them the two bowls of oatmeal, along with one small pitcher of hot milk. Dennie no longer wanted to start a conversation. She was hungry. The oatmeal was good. She devoured it. Kim looked at hers.

107

"Look, if you'd rather I came back some other day. . . ."

"What? Oh. No. Today is fine. Another day could be as bad. It's just that we just lost a kid. It's the first time that's happened to me. With a little kid, I mean. That's different from an adult. This was a six-year-old boy. He'd been hit by a car. We couldn't save him. It sort of. . . . It. . . . Well, it reminded me of my sister. I. . . ." She started to cry.

There was nothing Dennie could say. Sometimes crying was the right thing to do.

Kim took a handkerchief out of her white jacket and dabbed her tears and blew her nose. "Sorry," she said. "You wanted to talk about Austin Flint. You're a friend of Leslie English, you said."

Dennie was very glad that Kim had brought up the name.

"How is Leslie? I used to babysit for her. I haven't seen her in years and years."

"She's fine," Kim lied. The truth wasn't important yet.

"What would you like to know? Other than sometimes we lose patients? And that seems like more than sometimes."

That was a good question. One for which Dennie hoped she was prepared. "I really wanted to talk to you about Leslie."

"About Leslie? But I thought. . . ."

"You see," Dennie interrupted, "Leslie has been having some very frightening dreams."

"Dreams?" Kim was confused.

"Yes. And in them a number of names keep reappearing."

"You some kind of a shrink?"

"A psychologist. A grad student really. In psych at DePaul. Clinical psych." She was getting good at this. "We're doing research on sleep and dreams. And she's one of our subjects. So we're trying to figure out who those names belonged to. The names in her dreams. Who they were in her real life?"

"Sort of like detective work," Kim commented.

"Sort of, I guess. Some she can remember. Some she can't. She remembered you. Most of the others meant nothing to her."

"I was her babysitter off and on for a couple of years."

"You and your sister."

"Just me," firmly. Almost harshly. "My sister never liked to babysit."

"She also remembered Happy Felsch."

"Poor Happy. She killed herself."

"You're kidding!" Dennie said, feigning surprise.

"That must have been three or four years ago. Let me see. . . ." By now Kim had put the tragedy of her day behind her. Distracted by Dennie's questions. Or Leslie's problem. Or Happy's tragedy. Or all three.

Happy had OD'd. She'd taken a combination of pills. Sleeping pills. Antidepressants. Tranquilizers. Kim began to act the medical student and talk about drug interactions. About lethal doses. About mechanisms of action. She caught herself. This was not an oral exam in pharmacology. Some of the pills had apparently been hers. Some had been her mother's. Most. It hadn't been a gesture.

A gesture?

A suicidal gesture. Lots of kids and adults, too, for that matter, made suicidal gestures. Not ever intending to really kill themselves. But suicide-like acts. Gestures. To get attention. To show their need. Their desperation. To call out for help.

How?

Take a few sleeping pills. Not enough to do any harm. Three or four. And leave notes. Or make phone calls and wait around to be rescued. Or slit their wrists very superficially. Lots of blood. Dark venous blood, but never bright red arterial blood. Messy but not dangerous. The problem was that sometimes they miscalculated.

Miscalculated?

Kim nodded.

How?

"Take Tylenol. Most people figure it's pretty damn safe. It must be. You buy it over the counter. Off the shelf. How dangerous could it be? You take a handful and then let somebody find you. Off to the hospital. They pump your stomach and its all over. What's the big deal? The big deal is that it can destroy the liver."

"Oh, God."

"That's the problem with gestures."

"But that's not what happened to Happy?"

"No. Hers was not a gesture. Anything but. That had been her second try. The first had been a gesture. The second had been the real thing. She knew that her grandmother was out of town. She went there. To her grandmother's. She had a key. She let herself in. And took all those pills. In a place where no one would look for her."

How did Kim know all those details?

"Her mom and my mom are still close friends."

"I see."

"She told my mom everything. Everything but the truth."

"What truth?"

"Her dad abused her."

"What?!"

"We always thought she was a clumsy kid. Some kids are. Clumsy little Happy. Always with bruises. Or a broken arm. Or a leg. That SOB."

"When she got older, do you think he abused her sexually?" There was no point in beating around the bush.

"I've learned one thing on pediatrics," Kim announced.

"What's that?"

"They often don't wait until the kids get older."

"Christ almighty!" They! Not just Kroller. But others. They! No matter what she'd read. What she'd heard. Confronting it was still horrifying. They didn't wait. What a thing to have to learn.

"Try me on some other names." Kim said, obviously shifting the conversation onto a pleasanter subject.

Or would it be?

Leslie had been raped by her dad. Correction, stepfather. In some sort of ritual in which Mrs. Felsch participated. She'd been part of the coven. A witness. A participating witch. A truly wicked witch. Had Happy's dad also been there? Had Happy? Poor Happy. Poor abused Happy. Had she also been molested? In the same sort of ritual? By the same women? As part of the same coven?

Did her mother also make thirteen in her nightmares?

Dennie went over the list. Kim only recognized one other name. Risberg. That belonged to another little girl. She was probably about Leslie's age. Kim had been her babysitter once or twice. A cute blond. Edie Risberg. Edith. After Edith Piaf. Her mother was French. Her father was Swedish. And very blond. And very, very rich. Even by Glencoe standards.

What did he do?

He made money. Otherwise she had no idea. What did kids know? He wasn't a doctor. He was a mister. For all she knew he was a lawyer. Or into real estate. Or white slavery, she joked.

The joke fell very flat.

It was almost nine. Kim had to get to rounds. One patient had died. Life went on. Rounds went on.

Did Kim know where Paul Richardson's office was?

She did. It was in this building. The Rohe Tower. Suite 1400.

✳✳✳✳

Paul Richardson was not in his office. But Professor Richardson, according to the receptionist, was expecting her. That meant that she was welcome to go into his office and wait for him there. He was making rounds in the hospital, but he should be finished quite soon. It was probably as good a place to wait as any other, so she availed herself of the offer. There was a well-worn chair behind a large desk. And one other not so well-worn chair against one of the walls. She had to hang up the dirty white laboratory coat that was draped over the chair in order to sit down on it. The chair was next to the door and looked past a corner of the desk to the same view of the Chicago skyline she'd seen from the seventh floor, only better. More spectacular. She could see everything from the John Hancock Building with its twin rabbit ear-like TV antennas, or was that ears-like antennae, to the Sears Tower. And everything in between. What a view. She loved it. A wonderful succession of rooftops varying from sculpted masonry to mounted water towers, which were little more than overgrown barrels, to parking lots to ugly air-conditioning units to glass boxes or triangles or quadrangles or other sorts of multiangle, polyangles. Whatever. A history of twentieth century architecture at a glance.

The other two walls had low filing cabinets along them. The walls above the cabinets were covered with pictures. Photos of old men. Mostly nineteenth century photographs, intermixed with works of art. There were a few paintings. Some oils. Some acrylics. One that stuck out brightly was a small Paschke. It was not alone. There were several other imagist images. Dennie got up to take a closer look at the Paschke. Then the Wirsum. No wonder he and Ward were friends. There were also pictures of what appeared to be patients. Drawings. And photographs. The patients had neurologic disabilities of various sorts. Most of them were old. Both the subjects and the photos. She guessed that they were reproductions of old textbook illustrations. Then she saw a photograph of a woman. A young woman in her early twenties. She was naked above her burlap skirt. Well built. Very well built. But there was something on her breasts. Something. . . . Dennie looked closer. She was usually not one to look at other women's breasts. Neither out of interest nor jealousy. The something was a pin. No. Pins. Safety pins! She'd had safety pins stuck through her breasts. Pushed through her breasts!

Ugh!

Sadistic bastard!

Was this what the jerk liked?

He and that Tom Ward. Ward was a cop. And all cops were probably into that sort of thing. Confusing sex with violence and pain. What did Beth see in Mike? Did Mike. . . ? She winced.

"I see you are admiring my art," he said. It was Paul Richardson. Long white coat and all.

"Some of it."

He sat down behind his desk, a desk covered with piles of opened books, stacks of papers, various pieces of statuary, and one framed picture of which Dennie could see only the back. He looked at it intently. Probably a centerfold complete with pierced. . . . She stopped herself and sat down.

"I only like some of it myself," he said.

"Then why is it all hanging in your office?"

"A good question. Some I used to like and hope maybe I'll like again someday. And some my wife won't live with at home. And some are just part of my life. That," he said, pointing to a nineteenth century portrait of a man in his sixties, "is George Huntington. He invented Huntington's chorea. Not really. But in sort of the same way Columbus discovered America. He didn't describe the disease for the first time, but he described it so well that others could recognize it from his description and diagnose it. The patients now had a specific disease. They had that chorea described by that American. By George Huntington. Huntington's chorea. It was the first American disease. Put America on the map of world medicine."

Why, she wondered, was he telling her all this? She wasn't a medical student. He knew why she was here. She wanted to talk about witchcraft.

"Huntington's families," he continued, "the families he studied, lived up in the Hamptons on Long Island. And they came from England. In 1830 with John Winthrop. Settled in Massachusetts. Good ol' Massachusetts. The cradle of our democracy. Plymouth Rock. Paul Revere. The Boston Tea Party. And Salem."

"Salem?"

"At least one witch had Huntington's chorea. She twitched. She danced. That's what chorea means—dance-like movements. The Groton witch. To her judges those dance-like movements of hers proved that she was possessed by the devil. Ergo, she was a witch."

"What started it all?" she asked.

"Those girls who made the accusations were also victims of sorts. Of a mass hysteria."

"But why witchcraft?"

"You have to remember the era. The times. They believed in witches. In England, the England they had left, it was a religious duty to seek out and kill witches. And everyone agreed on two things. Both the Church of England and the nonconformists. The Puritans. No, three things. Witches were real. They existed. They had secret compacts with the devil himself. And they had to be rooted out and destroyed.

"In England witch-hunters canvassed the countryside. They got twenty shillings from the government for every suspected witch who was jailed.

Suspected witch," he repeated. "All that was needed was the accusation, not conviction. Once that happened the witch-hunters could receive their rewards. What a system. Just like Joe McCarthy. No proof required. Just a name on a list of names. Witchcraft was their form of communism. A deadly sin. So what happened? What always happens? Hundreds of odd or strange or merely unpopular people were tortured and executed. Thousands. As witches. As enemies of humanity. Maybe blacklisting wasn't so bad."

Richardson continued his discussion. It was more than she wanted from him, but she didn't stop him. The fundamental beliefs about witchcraft in the New England colonies were pretty much the same as those in England. This was not yet the America of Thomas Jefferson. And George Washington. Ben Franklin. It was the America of Cotton Mather.

"What happened?"

"Witch-hunts. What else? Each witch scare began in the same way. It always started with a woman. Often some old woman. A widow. A displaced person. One of the homeless of that era. That woman would be accused of having taken on spectral changes in her appearance and actions. The specific changes varied from witch to witch. From town to town. From accuser to accuser. But they were all the same. The woman had consorted with Satan himself. The woman gave her body and soul to the devil and had forsaken God and the church."

"And they believed all that?"

"They were all good religious people. God-fearing. Good Christians all. They had read their Bible."

"Do people still believe in witches?"

"The Church still does. Of course, they just figured out that Galileo hadn't committed heresy when he said the sun didn't circle the earth. Justice sometimes moves very slowly."

"But today?" Why did he digress so? "Are there witches?"

"People possessed by the devil? That's not a scientific question. That's a matter of faith."

"No, I mean, are there witches?"

"Cults of witches? Is that what you mean?"

"Yes."

"Covens? Sure. They're usually called satanic cults."

"Do they cause psychiatric problems?"

"Wait a minute. Do you mean are they caused by psychiatric problems? Or do they cause them in others?"

"Cause them in others."

"Who?"

"Victims. Children."

"It's generally thought so. I have some papers here. Somewhere in this mess," he said, gesturing vaguely with both arms. Very vaguely. "I might be able to find them," he added, not very hopefully. "You might run a Medline search."

"I already did that," proudly.

"Then you know there's a whole literature on the subject."

"Three papers."

"Only three?" He seemed to be genuinely surprised. "Not exactly a whole literature."

"Why not?" she asked.

"You know much of that is either in the psychoanalytic literature. Or postanalytic. Neoanalytic. Non-Freudian. Freud didn't believe in witches. Jung did. All that cultural unconscious mumbo jumbo. Symbols. Dragons. Witch's hats. Swastikas. All that crap."

"So?"

"That literature moves very slowly. In science a paper delayed means progress forestalled. In Jung? Ha! What difference does it make? So it takes years for papers to be published. And besides, they believe in the oral tradition."

"The oral tradition?"

"They have meetings and tell each other their stories. So they all know what's going on. But they never get published."

"So they're not in Medline."

"You got it. Neither are most chapters in most books. And analysts are big on books that get sold to lots of nonphysicians."

"Like John Doran."

"Who?"

"A psychologist in town."

"The town's full of them."

"He believed in witches."

"I doubt that."

"What do you mean?"

"He might well believe that there are covens of witches. And that kids are hurt by them. There is a literature on that. Witches as a cause of multiple personalities. And depression. Suicide. And he might even treat such patients. But that doesn't mean he believes in witches. Unless he is very Jungian."

"He was very Jungian."

"Was?"

"He's dead. He was murdered."

"By a stake in the heart?" Paul inquired facetiously.

"A knife in the back. A butcher knife."

"More reliable. Those stakes never worked. They were wooden. Too thick to do the job."

They both fell silent.

"You know, our beliefs change over time. What used to be true isn't anymore. And vice versa. Take Saint Joan."

"Saint Joan?"

"No one doubted that she heard voices. And it was never a question of her sanity. Did she hear voices? Was she crazy? Were they merely hallucinations? No. She heard voices. No question about it.

"But whose voice? That was the question. God's voice. Or. . . ?" he paused. "Or the devil's? That was all that had to be decided. So a decision was made. Undoubtedly more on political than religious grounds, true. But a decision. She was burned as a heretic. A witch who consorted with the devil."

She was beginning to understand.

"It's like beauty," he went on.

"Beauty?"

"In the eye of the beholder. Did you notice that woman, the one in the burlap skirt?"

"Is that what you think is beautiful? A woman with safety pins pushed through her breasts?"

"Those Victorians had all the fun," he complained.

"Fun!" angrily.

"They did that to show that she was hysterical. She felt them touch her breasts but she did not feel the pinpricks."

"Those pricks!"

He ignored her epithet. "They believed in hysteria. As a common disease. And they didn't know that a neurologic problem could cause loss of pain sense without causing any loss of touch. To the Church of Saint Joan's day, that would have been proof that she had suckled the devil. Off with her head. Or burn her at the stake. To early psychiatrists and neurologists, it was a classic case of hysteria. To us, a specific neurologic disease."

Thank God he wasn't into safety pins. She reached over to his desk and turned the picture around. It was the woman from the gallery in a formal gown.

"My wife," he said. "She was at the Wadsworth show. You didn't meet her. She's a . . . ," he paused, ". . . the best."

"I know."

"What are those Jungian meetings like?" she asked. "I picture them as something like the convention of wizards that the Wizard of Oz was going to attend."

"To hobnob with his fellow wizards?"

"Yes."

"I think of them more as a convention of village idiots. But you may be right. Village idiots are more innocent than wizards. Tell me, where do you go from here?"

"I'll read these three articles. And then I'll talk to the people at the Jung Institute."

"Ask them a question for me," Paul requested. "Ask them how they can take Jung seriously."

"What do you mean?"

"The SOB was a nazi!"

"What?"

"A nazi. And he was Swiss. He joined up because he wanted to. He believed all that Aryan superior race b.s. A nazi. You ask them how can they believe in symbolism that ends up in that kind of behavior?"

"I will," she said. She, too, had a question. "What happened to the Cardinal who said Joan was a heretic?"

"And the Pope who let her get burned at the stake?" he added. "They must be burning in hell. But only if."

"If what?"

"If you believe in hell."

Polygons. She'd remembered. Polygonal shapes. And Popes burning in hell. Detective work was fun.

"One other thing. There is someone else who might be able to help you."

"Who?"

"One of my associates. Her name is Kris Swensen. She's read a lot about modern witchcraft. She's out of town today. Some meeting. I'll ask her to give you a call."

"Thanks, and thanks for all the help."

Chapter
X

Tom Ward arrived on time and armed with half a dozen bagels, two each of plain, onion, and pumpernickel. He had not known her long enough to know which sort of bagel she preferred. One didn't get to such personal issues so early in a relationship. And he had also brought all the trimmings. Cream cheese, lox, a large tomato, and a Bermuda onion. She sliced both the tomato and the onion while he cut the bagels and put the lox on a plate.

"Coffee?" she inquired.

"No. Of course not. I brought cream soda."

"What's that?" she asked.

"A sort of pop. It goes with cream cheese and lox. It's a New York tradition. Cream pop."

"But you're not from New York." A statement, not a question.

"How do you know?"

"To a New Yorker, 'pop' means Dad. They all say 'soda.' Cream soda. Never cream pop. That's Chicago. Right out of Mayor Daley's Southside. The real Mayor Daley."

"You'd make a great detective."

"Not me. Beth's the real detective in the family. Compared to her, I'm a dilettante. She's the one who taught me. . . ." Dennie had made a mistake and she knew it and there was no way to go back. She just stopped, hoping he would not pursue it. She made herself a sandwich. A pumpernickel bagel. Lox, cream cheese, a slice of tomato. But no onion. She hoped he'd follow suit. He didn't. He put a thick slice of onion on his. A very thick slice.

"You want to show me yours first?" she asked.

He did and said so without so much as a single double entendre. Some days were like that.

His tape was hard to make out. The camera remained focused on the couch. The lighting was so dim that the couch was little more than a vague shape. And, of course, it had no introductory titles and no narration. A few voices in the background were all that she could make out.

"It goes on like this for half an hour or so," he explained.

"Gripping drama," she quipped. "The script is not much. Sort of out of Pinter by way of Beckett, but the cinematography is brilliant. Worthy of Bergman."

"I get it." He pushed FAST FORWARD. And finally the image on the screen changed. Not the background. The couch did not move. God, she was sick of that couch. Then something entered the foreground. A shape. Big. Round. Black. Tom hit PLAY. The shape came into sharper focus. It was the back of a bald head. A bald black head. Of the bald head of a black. A black male. A big black male. The head turned, giving them a side view. A profile complete with thick neck.

That neck. It was that same neck. And that same profile. The face turned. Into the camera.

It was that face.

That cop.

"He's a cop," she said. "He confronted me at Doran's office."

"He's not a cop," Tom told her. Somehow she was not completely surprised. "His name is Eller. Scott Eller. He and his brother work for Kroller as bodyguards."

"I met his brother, Horace. At Kroller's. He's one big guy."

"So is Scott."

"Is bodyguard a euphemism?" she asked.

"Isn't it always?"

"For goon?"

"More or less."

Scott Eller's face was now staring at the camera from less than two feet away. One foot. Curiously. With his nose getting too big for his face. Angrily.

"SHIT!"

The face yanked itself out of the field.

"He knows," Tom said.

"What?"

"That we know."

"What was he doing?" she asked.

"Looking around," noncommittally.

"For what?"

"You tell me."

"Leslie's videotapes."

"Perhaps. But why?"

"So that Kroller could find out just what she'd said to Doran."

"They had her deposition. She can't say anything in court that wasn't said in her deposition."

"But she remembers more on those tapes than she does by herself."

"What do you mean?"

She explained. Sipping away on her cream soda. It would never replace diet A & W root beer. She told him about the list of names. The twelve witches. Leslie had remembered them during a session with Doran. It hadn't been easy. Not like reciting the names of the months. But she remembered them all. It was almost as if she were in some sort of trance. As if she were really into her memories. But when Dennie had asked her about the witches, Dennie had to read her the list. It was almost as if she were mesmerized.

"Mesmerized?" Tom asked, unfamiliar with the term.

"Hypnotized. Mesmer invented hypnosis."

"Hypnotized."

"Yes. I guess that's what therapy is all about. A mindset that allows you to remember more."

"So maybe Eller was after Leslie's tape."

"Don't sound so convinced," Dennie commented. She was not quite sure how to make this man out. He was hard to read. "Sean may use these tapes at trial," she added.

Tom was still unimpressed. "Tell me about that list."

She did. From Collins to Berger. So far she'd been able to account for six of twelve. Five Leslie had remembered. One Kim Williams had added.

Who was Kim Williams?

A medical student who used to babysit for Leslie.

Leslie had a medical student as a babysitter?

Of course not. She told him the entire story. From Leslie to Kim to Edie. Edie Risberg. Named Edith after Piaf. One of them had committed suicide.

One of the twins?

No. Not one of the twins. One of the other witch's kids.

One of the witches?

Happy.

A happy witch?

Happy Felsch.

Tom was lost. She had been moving too fast, covering too much territory too quickly. She started over and told him everything she knew. The words tumbled out in a torrent. She again told him about Kim Williams and her little sister. And Happy Felsch. Everything she knew. He listened carefully until she was done.

"Another deal," he said once she came up for air.

"What's that?"

"A proposition. I'll check out the other names with Mrs. Kroller for you. You stay away from the Krollers. I don't trust them. Mrs. Kroller ought to know some of those names. She has to. They have to be names from the past of the Kroller family. All twelve of them. If they were in that craven."

"Coven," she corrected him. "A witches' coven."

"That's what I said. The coven involved Mrs. Kroller and her neighbors and friends. Sort of a block club. So I'll check out Mrs. Kroller. I'll also check out that Williams kid."

"Kim?"

"Her dead sister."

"It was an accident."

"Are you sure of that?"

She wasn't sure of anything. Except that she was scared. This was not a game. Someone had been murdered. And had tried to kill her. Sometimes she could ignore all that. Other times she couldn't. This was one of those other times. She bit her lip hard. What was she supposed to do as her part of his proposition?

"Keep following up the names on the list. The ones Leslie English remembered."

That sounded fair to her. These names were probably herrings. Red herrings couldn't hurt her. Or blind alleys. Red herrings sounded a lot safer.

"I've shown you mine," he reminded her.

That meant that it was time for her to show him hers. A deal was a deal. She put on one of the tapes from Doran's office. It was not one that she had seen before. The patient was a very frightened young woman named Rowe. Nancy Rowe. She seemed to be about seventeen years old at the most. Maybe younger. Sixteen. In high school. A schoolgirl.

A schoolgirl who was frightened.

Of what?

Of men. Of boys.

All men? All boys? Doran led her through her recital. Was it all men? All boys? All males? Or one particular male? As always, Doran knew where to probe. What to pursue. What to ask.

One particular male, she conceded.

Which one?

Her father. It was all so damn familiar. A familiarity that bred fear. And loathing. And nausea. Overwhelming nausea.

Once again Doran took the lead. Just her father?

No.

Who else?

Women.

All women?

The same scenario. With the same outcome. She was afraid of her mother. Under Doran's guidance, Nancy began to relax. To lose her fear. To get beyond it. Behind it and as she did she began to remember more.

He was certainly good at what he did.

Nancy began to remember. To describe her memories. To relive them. As if they were still happening. Memories of a past life that was not past. Not gone. Alive. A part of her mind and soul. Happier times. Childhood times. Games. Fun. Dances. Dances around a fire. A bonfire. That sounded right. A bonfire. With her mom. And other women.

And other women.

How many other women?

She couldn't remember.

She would. Soon. And that would help her. Remembering always helped.

If only that were true, Dennie thought to herself. If only that were true.

The second patient on the tape did not have a name. Only a letter. B.

She was black. And in her late thirties or early forties. With short hair. Short and very curly.

"Hi," she said, lying down on the couch. "I'm B. I'm twenty-four."

"And I'm sixteen," Dennie countered.

"I'm thirty-eight," B. went on.

That seemed closer to the truth.

"Thirty-eight, twenty-six, thirty-six."

That seemed possible. Although she looked heavier around the middle. More than twenty-six. Every woman was allowed some degree of latitude. Of hyperbole. If that was the right word.

"Thirty-eight D." And with that B. started to unbutton her dress. Slowly. Starting at the top. One button at a time. All the time making certain to keep her dress closed. From top to bottom. Then just as slowly, no, more slowly, she began to let the dress edge open. Again in the same direction. From top to bottom. Revealing her chocolate-brown flesh.

D seemed no exaggeration. Pushing out above a black bikini bra. Very black. Jet black.

Then came more chocolate. A waist that was a couple of inches more than twenty-six. And bikini panties. Again black. Jet black. She patted herself on those black panties. And then rubbed herself softly several times. "Black is beautiful," she said. And with a shrug the entire dress disappeared below her.

She licked her lips. They became wetter. And redder. And far more alive. The color contrasts came out quite well, despite the limited lighting. The redness of the lips on that couch reminded Dennie of the first image she had seen of Doran. With bright red blood at the base of a butcher knife. Could this woman have wielded that knife?

She reached behind herself and the bra almost flew off of her.

D.

At least. With long, thick, dark nipples. She cupped her breasts, aiming them at the unseen camera.

Did she know about the camera? Dennie was willing to bet that she did. And was playing to that camera. Not remotely.

Then she shifted a bit. Bent her knees. Wiggled her hips. Lifted them. And the panties were gone.

Another pat. In the same place. But the panties were no longer there. This time her hand was patting a thick patch of blue-black hair. Her knees and hips remained bent. Then her knees began to fall away from each other ever so slowly.

Then they started undulating. Sideways. Back and forth. "When did I start?"

"Yes, when did you start?" John Doran asked. A rather straightforward question. And clearly directive.

"Fucking?"

"Fucking for money." Very directive.

"Same time. Same day," she chuckled. "Same fuck."

"Tell me about it." Extremely directive.

She had been twelve. It was her brother's birthday. He had two of his friends staying over for the night. They didn't want to be bothered by her. They wanted to play poker. She wanted to play, too. She could only play on one condition. What was that? They'd play strip poker.

"Some client," Dennie said.

"But who is the client?"

Dennie wasn't sure what Tom meant.

Soon everyone had lost. But no one wanted to stop playing. And they had been playing for money.

She didn't have any money.

Her brother knew what they could play for.

"Enough," Tom said, turning off the tape.

"What did you mean?"

"Enough is enough."

"Pretty personal stuff."

"No. Not personal at all."

"Not personal at all? What do you want, an exact description of her brother's prick? Whether he was circumcised or not? That poor little girl. Conned into a gang rape at age twelve. No wonder she needs to see a shrink."

"I'm sure she does."

"I'm sure she's devastated that Doran is dead. She'll have to start all over. To tell that whole ugly story to someone else. Again. To start all over. Poor girl."

"That poor girl tells that story for a living."

"What?"

"She's a hooker. A pro. A. . . ."

"I know what a hooker is," she said angrily. This cop was one grade A callous bastard. She wondered what he had done to his sister? To his wife? No wonder she divorced him. It had probably been a no-fault divorce. And one hundred percent of the no-fault was his. Jackass!

"And her so-called therapist was the client. Not Bea. Doran. He paid her. This had to be how he got his kicks."

"I don't believe that."

"Let's take a look." He got up and walked into the kitchen and then into Beth's apartment.

"If she's a hooker, it's because of what her brother made her do to him. That little fucker," she yelled after him. Men.

He was back. With a copy of *The Reader.* It was a recent issue.

"What are you doing?"

"I'm reading the personals."

"The personals?"

"Adult services." He handed her a page.

She scanned it. She had never done this before. There were hundreds of ads. Ads for phone sex. Of every variety. Lesbian. Gay. Straight. Transsexual. You name it. She couldn't name any others. The services could. A lot of others. She moved on to the next column. Massage services.

"Massage is a euphemism for. . . ."

"I know," she interrupted him. She hadn't been born yesterday.

Massage services. Female masseuses. Male masseurs. Transsexual. Now there was a real conundrum. Was a transsexual a masseuse or a masseur? More females. Brandy. Sabrina. The first had red hair. The second didn't. Tracy. Christine. B.

B.

She handed the page to Tom Ward. He had been the one who had wanted to prove that B. was a whore. Well, he'd proven that to her. But why was she a hooker? Because she'd been gang-banged by her brother and his friends at age twelve. Her own brother. That was the cause.

He dialed the number listed in the ad.

B. answered.

It was the same voice that had been on John Doran's video.

He'd called about the ad.

"I'm twenty-four," she began.

The exact same voice. With the exact same lie.

"I'm thirty-eight. Thirty-eight, twenty-six, thirty-six. Thirty-eight D."

That was true. The D part at least.

"A nude massage costs one hundred bucks."

Ward asked if that included a full body massage?

It did.

"Do you do. . . ?"

"I do what pleases. For extra."

"Do you tell stories?"

"What kind of stories?"

"Sexy stories."

"Sure. For fifty more."

"About your first time."

"Why not?"

"With your father?"

"Father was best."

Tom hung up the phone.

"Dirty old man," she chided him, trying to make light of what he had said but being none too successful.

"Yes," distractedly. "We may have to see all of Doran's tapes. Every single one of them."

"Why?"

"What if he had a tape of some semipro."

"A semipro?"

"That's someone. . . ."

"I know what a semipro is. Like John Johnston."

"Who?"

She told him about John Johnston. He was a client of Doran's who gave full body massages to men as a hobby.

"Let me see the tape," he told her. Very officially. Then added, "we have to be sure who the client was."

She got the video from her shelf and put it in the VCR and pushed PLAY.

On came the image of the couch again. The couch on which John Doran had been knifed. Then the credits. Then John Johnston.

"That's him," she screamed. "The guy who saved my life. The lawyer."

"Who?" Tom was lost.

She told him the story of the attempt on her life. The cement bucket. The push. The near miss. The cracked sidewalk. From beginning to end. Except for Beth's phone call. Even the part about the dude. The black dude. The goon. The goon she had not seen.

"And he pushed you out of the way?"

"It was almost as if he were expecting something to happen."

"Perhaps he was."

"Why? How?"

"His name's not Johnson."

"Not Johnston?"

"Not that either."

"What is it?"

"Kroller."

"Kroller as in our Kroller?"

"As in our Kroller. His son. By his first marriage. Leslie's half brother. William Kroller, Jr. "Little Billie.""

"He's not her half brother. He's her stepbrother. Kroller never adopted her. There is a difference."

That wasn't the point. He was a semipro and Doran had proof of that. Maybe that was what Eller was after. The tapes of John Johnston. Of Billie Kroller. Not of Leslie English.

The tapes!

"John figured out about the tapes," she suggested.

"Maybe."

"He did. You can see that at the end of his session. At least I think you can. Maybe he got angry and then maybe he killed Doran."

"He couldn't have," Tom told her. "He was in the closed psych unit at Austin Flint. He signed back in at seven thirty. Doran was killed at around ten."

"He was out yesterday when he saved my life."

"Are you sure it was him?"

"Yes."

"Then why didn't you recognize him?"

"He had on a hat. And a muffler. And glasses. And a mustache. And I just wasn't paying any attention. It was cold and wet and windy. And we were both in a hurry to get cabs."

"We'll have to talk to this Billie Kroller. Mr. William Kroller, Jr.," Tom concluded.

"We?"

"Yes. Lieutenant Tom Ward and Deputy Sheriff Cater."

Tom knew. That guy must have been a cop. "When?" she asked.

"I'll call you later," he said, and then he added, "and be very careful."

"Professional advice?"

"Personal."

"I will," she said.

"They probably got what they wanted from you."

"What was that?"

"The keys to Doran's office."

"Then why the cement bucket?"

"I'm not sure," he informed her.

"And how did Kroller get out to save me?"

"I don't know."

"Why did he save me?"

"Maybe he'd gotten what he wanted. The key. Maybe that was all he wanted from you. That was enough to satisfy him."

"But not someone else?" she asked. She was getting more frightened. Talking about it made it more real. Someone had tried to kill her. And might again. She had to think about something else. Something less frightening. Something less threatening. Something that would make her feel less alone. Something. Someone. "Have you gotten enough to be satisfied?"

"Have you?" he countered.

"I asked first," she reminded him.

"No."

"Me neither."

She walked over and kissed him. His lips tasted of lox. So did his teeth. And his tongue. As well as onion. And cream cheese. She pressed against him.

"I'm not thirty-eight," she said.

"No, you're only twenty-eight."

He knew her exact age. But that wasn't what she'd meant. "Not D."

"C is okay."

"Will you settle for B?"

"Of course, but I've got to go," he said, pulling away just as she was beginning to sense that he was responding to her. Some days are like that.

"I'll call you later," he promised.

"You'd better."

"Dennie, I won't play games with you. Please don't play games with me."

"I won't," she promised. "Believe me. I won't. I'm too scared to play games." If only that were true.

✳✳✳✳

The Jung Institute of Chicago was on North Michigan Avenue. Not the real North Michigan Avenue. Not the Magnificent Mile, stretching north from the Chicago River and the site of the original Fort Dearborn that had not survived the Indian Massacre of 1807, past the original Water Tower that had survived the Chicago Fire, to the Oak Street Beach. A mile occupied by Saks, Marshall Field, Gucci, and Bloomie's. The Magnificent Mile. It was on the other part of North Michigan. South of Fort Dearborn. The wrong side of the Chicago River. With record stores. Discount importers. Video outlets.

The receptionist gave her no trouble at all. The director would be happy to talk to her. That was what he did. Lots of people came in looking for help and asking about Jungian therapists. His job was to explain the Jungian approach and help them find a good therapist. A good, Jungian therapist. The way she said that made it seem as if the two adjectives made up a redundancy.

The director was in his early forties. Thin. Balding. Wire-rimmed glasses. And a fetish for order. Not a hair was out of place. Nor a book. Each one was in its place, exactly one inch from the front of the bookshelf. The pictures were all precisely level. And so were the dozen or more diplomas. So many diplomas. One was a Ph.D. from somewhere in Switzerland. The others were from all over, including some from Florida. Doran had had identical certificates.

"Dr. Slaughter," she began.

"Slatter," he corrected her, with a trace of an accent. A Germanic accent. "Dr. Slatter. I'm Swiss. From Basle. Jung was also from Basle."

"I'm. . . ."

"I do not need to know your name. Just the general nature of your inquiry." Very precisely said.

"I have these dreams," she began, settling down into the chair across his desk from him. The desk was made of black iron with a glass top. On it was a single magazine. And a black lamp. And a black telephone.

"Dreams," he echoed her last word. He had studied Adler as well as Jung. Under the glass table he crossed his legs at the ankles. His hands rested flatly on top of the glass. Palms down. Passive. Immobile. More a stoic inquisitor than a therapist.

"Terrible dreams," she continued, portraying more than just a touch of distress. "Frightening. Scary. They really frighten me. And I don't know where they come from."

"That is often the case," he said knowingly.

"Or what they mean," with an added touch of desperation and urgency, trying not to be overdramatic.

"That is what we are for," he said, finally changing his posture. Not much but enough so that his left palm came to rest on his right wrist.

She shifted uncomfortably, crossed her right leg over her left leg at the knee, exposing her entire right calf and a part of her right thigh, and began to kick her right leg nervously, rhythmically, anxiously. Agitation, not panic. "So frightening. They wake me up. Every night. In a sweat. My nightgown is often drenched with sweat. Sometimes it's so wet I have to change nightgowns. In the middle of the night."

"Yes," promptingly.

Enough prologue, he was interested in details. "It . . . the dreams . . . the dream. It's always the same dream, or it seems so to me. The same terrible dream. I'm in the middle of a circle. A circle of . . . of women. Old women, I think. But I'm not an old woman. I'm not a woman. I'm a girl. A young girl. It's me. Me as a child. I'm five years old. Maybe six. It doesn't matter, does it?"

"Probably not," he paused before leading her on. "The women?"

"They're women. Older, maybe in their thirties and forties and even older. And bigger. So much bigger. And . . . and they look like witches. There, I've said it. I've never said it before. Witches. These witches are dancing around a bonfire. Around me and a bonfire," she sobbed just once. There was no need to get completely carried away.

"How do you know they are witches?"

It was a good question. And she knew the answer. "It's their clothes. Their long gowns. Long black gowns. They are all wearing black gowns."

"Lots of women wear black. I'll bet that you do at times."

"Not long plain black gowns like those, and not . . . not . . . not those hats."

"What hats?"

"Witch's hats. Round. Pointed. Like big black upside-down ice cream cones. Witch's hats. They're all wearing witch's hats," hoping she had not overdone it as she kicked away nervously.

"How many women?"

"Lots."

"Try to remember."

She closed her eyes and stopped kicking. She reshifted her legs. Left on right. "Ten, at least ten."

"Do you recognize any of them?"

Should she? Now, before therapy? She had no idea. She started kicking her leg again. This time it was her left leg and even more thigh was exposed than before. "They all seem familiar. Like I ought to recognize them, but shouldn't I by now? I see them every night."

"Do you recognize any one of them?"

"No, I can't say that I do," she guessed. This time her nervousness wasn't entirely feigned.

"Good," he smiled. He actually smiled. It was a weak smile and lasted only a couple of seconds, but it was clearly a smile.

"Why is that good?" she pleaded.

"You are a wonderful candidate for therapy. It's all right there. Ripe to be harvested but not yet polluted. Pure. Virginal."

She frowned.

"Your dreams. No one else has manipulated them?"

"No. God, no. I've told no one else about them."

"Don't, until you get a therapist," he warned her.

"Do I need a therapist?"

"Isn't that why you are here?"

She shifted her legs again. More kicking. More thigh. "I . . . I . . . guess . . . I. Yes. Yes, I need help."

He recrossed his legs, showing a bit more sock.

It was her move. "But should it be a Jungian? I mean, shouldn't I just see a Freudian analyst? Like my friends do?"

"No. Not at all. Freud. And don't get me wrong. Freud was a genius. And pivotal. In the right place at the right time, with some of the right ideas. The primacy of the unconscious. The importance of dreams. But he didn't understand the meaning of symbols."

"Symbols?" Two could play that game of directive therapy.

"Like the witch's hat."

"The witch's hat?"

"To Freud that would have been a male sex symbol. Long, round, straight. All very phallic. But why a witch's hat?"

"Yes, why?"

"Because a witch's hat is a basic symbol built into our brains. Here, look." He handed her the magazine that was on his desk. It was not a magazine at all. It was an auction catalogue of antiquities from a Chicago antiquities and coin dealer named Harlan Berk. It was full of illustrations of antiquities. Greek bronzes, Egyptian statuettes, clay lamps from Israel.

"Turn to number 794."

She did. It was a witch. The bronze statue of a witch. Seven inches high with a two-inch pointed conical hat.

"It's from the Iberian peninsula. That's Spain. About one thousand B.C."

"A witch," she said.

"With a witch's hat. That's a universal symbol. It was part of early Aryan culture. It's built into our brains. An archetypal symbol. Freud never understood that. Jung did. He knew the fact that the witch's hat is already in our brain. That's why it's so frightening."

"Like a swastika."

"Yes."

"So that's why the church made the Jews wear witch's hats."

"Yes. Yes. Freud would never admit that. He was Jewish."

"Do lots of people dream about witches?" she asked.

"Yes. More than you'd think."

"I. . . . I tried to look it up in the library."

He waved his hand dismissively. "Useless. The analytic literature is controlled by Freudians. We are the only ones who understand witchcraft." Defensive. Angry.

"I heard about one therapist. A Dr. Dorman," she suggested.

"Doran."

"That's it. Doran."

"He's very good, but he is not available."

Not available. What a quaint way to put it. "Oh," disappointed.

"I'll give you three names." With that, he reached onto the shelf behind him, opened a polished wooden box, picked out three cards, and handed them to her. "They are all excellent therapists."

"As good as Doran?"

"Doran, ah, yes. And more available."

That was undoubtedly true. She thanked him and got up to leave, reached in her purse, and handed him her card.

"Three Sisters Limited," he read. "Chekhov?"

"Andrews."

"Who?"

"No matter. By the way, I heard a rumor that Jung was, well . . . was a nazi."

"Propaganda," he exploded. "Jewish lies. Freudian lies. Never. They can't attack the symbols. So they attack Jung. As if it were the nazis who invented powerful symbols. And anyone who liked symbols had to be a nazi. It's symbol envy. That's a Jungian joke."

"Sorry," she said. Although she certainly wasn't.

✳✳✳✳

On her way home she did some grocery shopping. She couldn't depend on Tom to supply every meal. While she was in the grocery she used the pay phone to call Sean Keneally. Had he heard from Elizabeth?

He hadn't. But he had heard from a certain Lieutenant Ward. He said that he wanted to talk to Elizabeth, although he called her Beth.

To arrest her?

No. She's a suspect. But no more than that. A suspect. One of several, he guessed. She should make sure that Elizabeth knew that.

She would.

Ward had also asked about her.

"What did you tell him?"

"Nothing much. You're my client. It's all privileged communication."

"Everything?"

"In my legal opinion. And I'm the lawyer."

She then called Mike at home, listened through the stupid Harry Carey baseball bit and left a message for Beth. Or for Mike to tell Beth. Beth was a suspect. One of many. Not a fugitive. Not a criminal. Dennie waited, hoping someone was there to pick up the phone. Hopefully Beth. No one did.

When she got home her answering machine was blinking at her. Beth, she hoped. It was Tom Ward. A very good alternative. They had an appointment to talk to William Kroller, Jr., alias John Johnston, at four, at Austin Flint, on the closed psych unit. That was on the eleventh floor of the Walsh building.

"Eleven Walsh at four P.M.," he repeated. "Be on time."

On time! She had only fifteen minutes. She put the milk in the refrigerator, left the rest of the groceries in the bags, and ran downstairs to grab a cab.

She got to Austin Flint at three fifty-five and to the Walsh building at three fifty-seven. To eleven Walsh at three fifty-nine. Not bad. Tom Ward was waiting for her opposite the elevators.

They exchanged polite greetings and Tom pushed the bell on the locked door. It was, she reminded herself, the locked unit.

There was no answer.

They waited.

Tom once again pushed the bell. It was really a buzzer. And they could hear it buzzing.

No response.

Another push. Longer.

Finally Tom knocked on the door in exasperation and shouted, "Police."

The door sprang open. "Thank God," the nurse said. "He's in 1108," she added.

"Who?"

"The guy who killed himself. Mr. Kroller." With that she turned and led them both to Room 1108. Tom went in first and then turned abruptly and pushed her out of the doorway.

"It's not pretty."

"I've seen dead bodies before."

"He took a gun and blew off the top of his head."

"How did he get a gun?"

"What do you mean?"

"This is a closed unit. With full suicide precautions, I'm sure. How did he get a gun?"

Tom had no answer to her question.

Chapter
XI

Dead! John Johnston was dead. My God. He'd killed himself. She'd just watched him on that tape. So alive. So angry.

Now he was dead. He had taken a gun and blown off the top of his head. That was what Tom had said. The top of his head. Exactly how had he done that? Had he inserted the gun into his mouth and waited for it to explode? She thought of the tape of John Johnston's other life. The life that he had described to John Doran from that couch in Doran's office the evening before Doran had been murdered. Maybe it was the other way around. It was an interesting possibility. Could it be that his life as Billie Kroller was his other life? That he was really John Johnston. That he had been! Male . . . whatever. No. He was William Kroller. Junior. The son of William Kroller. That man disgusted her. And frightened her. Had this been because of his father. Wasn't it always because of the father? Some sort of Oedipal battle. From Sophocles, out of Freud, by way of hell. Why not? No reason. But Dennie had no way to judge. What had Beth said on her tape? Doran could have been with a man. All it took was some imagination. Somehow she was certain that both John Doran and John Johnston had imagination enough. More than enough.

She shivered as she thought of Billie Kroller placing a gun, the long, hard barrel of a gun, into his own mouth. Obvious Freudian symbolism there.

Or was it Jungian? Pre-Freudian, so to speak. Archetypal. Phallic symbols long antedated Freud. And guns for that matter. So did mother goddesses. And witches. Covens of witches. Satanic rituals. She'd always thought of witches as anti-Christian. Anti-Catholic. Anti-church. Mocking the Mass. Black Masses. But if the symbols were archetypal, that was wrong. They were really pre-Christian. Primitive. A basic, built-in belief system. Just like Jung discovered.

Is that what Doran had believed? Or merely used, took advantage of, to help his patients? Believing in Satan was irrelevant. All the therapist was supposed to do was treat his patient. Believe in the patient. In Leslie.

Leslie! Poor abused Leslie. Doran's murder had set her adrift. She had to be suffering now. Leslie needed another therapist. And soon. Now. But who? Dennie had three names. Three more Jungian therapists. Maybe one of them could help Leslie just as much as John Doran had. As John Doran had helped so many others. As he had helped John Johnston? In psychiatry did you judge success by outcome? What else was there? What other gauge? By that gauge John Doran certainly had not helped Billie Kroller.

Was that why Billie had killed him? But had Billie killed him? In a rage? A homosexual panic? Why not?

Billie was dead. John Johnston was dead. But John Johnston had never been alive. It was Billie Kroller who was dead. William Kroller, Jr. The man who had saved her life. No one had ever saved her life before. No one else had ever had the opportunity. Would someone else have that same opportunity?

She shivered yet again and looked about the room. The nurse who had taken her to the room had called it a therapy room. It was small. Nine by eleven or twelve, she guessed. It had no windows. And was only sparsely furnished. There was one narrow couch on which she was seated. Doran's office had also had one couch. She had to stop perseverating on that couch. There were also a small desk and three chairs. All very plain. And austere. No book cases. No file cabinets. No artifacts of human history. No memorabilia of anyone's personal history. No picture of loved ones. Three of the walls each held one poor quality reproduction. All three were of Impressionist scenes. Neutral Impressionist scenes. Almost sterile in their prettiness. A haystack by Monet. As neutral as possible. Not tall enough to be phallic. A haystack as a haystack. Some flowers in a vase. No stamen. No pistil. Flowers. And certainly not by Georgia O'Keeffe. Nothing vaginal about them. No strong vulvar features. Nothing sexual at all. And a wheat field by van Gogh. A pastoral scene. Nice and safe. What could be more neutral than this room? Less threatening?

Then why did she feel so damn threatened?

The fourth wall consisted mostly of a mirror. A mirror that was four feet high and six feet wide. It wasn't a real mirror. Not to look into and see your own reflection. Your mirror image. Your racemic other half. It was a ceiling made of glass. Except it was a wall instead of a ceiling. And it wasn't plain glass. One-way glass. For someone else to see in. To watch. To observe. To dissect.

Was there a video camera behind there? Or merely a couple of chairs?

John Johnston had figured it out. He'd realized what was behind that small window in Doran's ceiling. But when? The evening of the murder. Why that day? Why then? Why not before?

Because he'd seen this room? Been in this room. This therapy room. Seen this mirror? Learned its purpose? Then when he saw that window above him. Above the couch in Doran's office. He saw it and figured it out. Doran had tapes of him. Audio or video? Video. For audio all you needed was a bug, a microphone. No window.

Doran had videotapes of him. Billie Kroller could have guessed that. Psychiatric insight. Revelation. But Doran didn't know who Billie really was. Doran had videotapes of a guy named John Johnston. Permanent videos. And some day he might realize that John Johnston wasn't John Johnston. That he was William Kroller, Jr.

That meant that Kroller could have killed John Doran.

He could have come back, seduced him, and killed him. And taken the tape of the killing. But not the others? Why not? Was he interrupted by Beth? Had she seen him? Was he trying to kill Beth?

Then why had he saved Dennie's life?

Thank God he'd happened to be there. It had been no accident. That cement bucket had not just happened to fall down toward her. It had been pushed. By a black dude. No accident at all. A sneak attack. As accidental as Pearl Harbor. And just as deadly. Thank God John Johnston had happened to be there.

Not John Johnston. William Kroller, Jr. The late Billie Kroller. And he had not just happened to be there. He'd been there to be there. To save her. Why? From whom? How had he known? What had he known?

She had no idea. These were questions that she could not answer. And they weren't fun. And now he was dead. Both of him.

From whom had he saved her?

William Kroller. That sure as hell seemed like the best answer to that question. He molested little girls. And had goons who tried to kill people. And a son who was a gay hooker and killed himself. Just your average everyday family man who was into a lot of businesses with cash flow. Like liquor, videos. Prostitute. . . . The word forced its way from the back of her throat into her consciousness. What business had more cash flow than prostitution? One hundred percent cash. No charges. No credit cards. No returns. No matter how dissatisfied the customer. The perfect business for someone who raped little girls.

The door opened.

"Tom," she gasped expectantly.

It wasn't Tom. It was the nurse. She looked in and smiled automatically.

"Company," she said, with obviously false enthusiasm.

And in walked William Kroller. Senior. And his wife. The Ice Maiden. Both looked distraught. Not in mourning. Not sad. No tears. Just anger.

"You bitch," he said to Dennie. No polite euphemisms for him. In a way Dennie liked that.

"William," his wife said, "we must control ourselves." Then turning to her, "You must forgive him. Billie was his only son. He is heartbroken."

Maybe he was.

"Bitch," he repeated.

Maybe not.

"This is all your fucking fault. Why don't you get the hell out of here? And out of my life? Before it's too damn late."

For whom? Wasn't it too damn late already for Billie?

"Something could happen to you."

"Something already has," she replied, remarkably calmly.

"If something had happened, you wouldn't be here, and . . . and. . . ." He was crying. What appeared to be real tears. And his wife put her arms around him. She was hugging him. Holding him tightly. Cradling his head to her shoulder. Not to her breast. There were limits to miracles.

It was a scene of grief. Of normal grief and human tragedy. A scene that seemed to be genuine. She felt uneasy watching it play itself out. It was time for her to go. Dennie looked at them, said "I'm sorry about your son," and walked out of the therapy room. She found the nurse.

"I've got to go someplace else. They need to be alone."

"I understand, but all the other treatment rooms are in use. So many patients have gone bonkers."

"I don't need treatment."

"You mean you just want to leave?"

"Yes."

"Without seeing your therapist?" the nurse asked.

"I don't have a therapist."

"You don't?" in abject disbelief.

"No, I don't."

That being the case, there was no reason not to let her go. As the nurse unlocked the outer door, Dennie asked her to give a message to Tom Ward. The police lieutenant. "Tell him that Deputy Cater is in the library."

✳✳✳✳

The library turned out to be easy to find. As was the article she wanted to read on witchcraft as a cause of multiple personalities. Had Billie Kroller actually had multiple personalities? Or merely two names? A name and an alias. Billie Kroller also known as John Johnston. AKA. Not a psychiatric disorder, but a disguise. A pseudonym. As innocent as Samuel Clemens and Mark Twain. Well, not quite that innocent. But just a second assumed name. Like so many hookers did. Was Bea "B."? What was her real name? Her real persona? Jill? Who had gone up the hill with Jack and come down pregnant. Or with VD. Not two personalities. Two names. There was a difference.

To work. No more stream of consciousness. There were articles she had to read. Articles on the role of witchcraft in causing psychiatric disorders. That issue, it seemed, was a matter of much debate. Both as to its role as a cause of a specific psychiatric disorder, and especially multiple personality disorder, and as a cause of any kind of psychiatric problem at all. Any kind of behavioral disorder. How could that ever be a question?

The critical issue, she learned, was the very basic question of credibility. What the hell did that mean? Did people doubt that they were telling the truth? Why would they lie?

In the past such patients had rarely been believed by their therapists. Very, very rarely, Freud hadn't believed his patients. Women had told Freud these stories. He had refused to believe them. Why should others? The women told their stories of sadistic abuse, of incestuous rape, of all sorts of incest, of pregnancy, of being locked in closets, or of being half buried. Their tales of horror were interpreted as fantasy. Or delusion. Or wish fulfillment. That was the one she liked best. Was that because most of them were women? Women who had been little girls? Little girls who had been raped by their fathers and had to seek help from other older men? Whose wish was being fulfilled? That sure as hell was the question.

These patients were not easy to help. They often had trouble getting in touch with their own feelings. They seemed to be dissociated from their own emotions. They often seemed to distort reality. Dissociation. Perceptual distortion. Dennie was really getting into the terminology. It was almost like being in grad school. She read about their dissociation and their perceptual distortions, their heightened longing for parents, and the recurring wish that the abuse had never occurred. At times the patients even accepted the skepticism of their therapists. The skepticism. And the disbelief. The rejection of that reality. The therapists didn't believe that they had been raped. Perhaps they hadn't been. They hadn't been. A real perversion of wish fulfillment. The rapes became dissociated memories. Something that had happened to someone else. Their so-called memory of abuse was a sign of their own pathology.

Wasn't psychiatry great? Poof, there goes child abuse. No more incest.

There was a reference to another paper, written in 1985. By Doran. J. Doran. Leslie's J. Doran. Doran had not challenged his patients' stories. He had a different approach. He believed them. He said that it helped. Others disagreed.

Over the years some real data had been accumulating. Child abuse became reportable in the mid-1960s and sexual abuse in the mid-1970s. The numbers grew by leaps and bounds. The severity of associated physical and emotional damage could no longer be ignored. Some therapists started to consider the possibility that even the extreme and bizarre accounts of sadistic torture in childhood might be true. Maybe the patients weren't lying. But remembering the truth. What was needed was independent confirmation. That sounded so cold. So legal! Sean had used the same phrase. Independent confirmation.

Of incestuous rape!

But it wasn't easy. The patients needed help to uncover their stories. Like Leslie. She had been able to reconstruct her story. But only with John Doran's help. She hardly even remembered the names of the witches by herself.

Why? As she read more and more, Dennie began to understand better. Leslie had tried to dissociate herself from the horror of it all. The horror! The abject horror.

Fucking bastard! To do that to a little girl.

That all seemed reasonable to Dennie. So what was the problem?

Patients like Leslie described ritual abuse. They told of scenes of satanic worship. Those scenes were so bizarre. So primitive. Out of a time long past. Most therapists just refused to believe them. This had to be fantasy or delusion. Not the resurfacing of dissociated memories of what had happened. These images were so alien to normal experience. Patients and therapists alike had trouble believing the stories. Unless the patient was suffering from psychosis. With a crazy story like that they had to be crazy. St. Joan on Freud's couch.

But not to Jungian therapists.

Not John Doran. He did not think that way.

What was Leslie going to do without him?

According to some authority named Heinrich Weber, several kinds of efforts were being made to supply a data base for ritual abuse. Therapists were now collecting accounts from many different victims so that they could begin to recognize typical patterns of such satanic abuse.

And one aspect of the satanic ritual experience was becoming very clear. The descriptions were often similar. The memories, no matter how distorted, how dissociated, followed a pattern. The pattern of a specific ritual. Of course. That's what made them rituals. Rituals were the same. The Mass didn't change. Nor did other rituals.

Most of the children were abused in the same way. As part of the same satanic ritual. With only minor variations. The use of the local language. That didn't change the Mass. Same order. Same meaning.

Same symbols.

Then why didn't their therapists believe them?

Because they were men? The altar of the witchcraft ritual was always a woman. She was the centerpiece. A naked woman. A naked woman with her legs spread apart. Far apart. A naked woman whose vagina would be penetrated. Reading the description made her feel that she too had been violated in the same way. That all women had been. Penetrated unwillingly.

And then the little girls whose. . . .

Sadistic bastards.

The article ended.

She needed to know more. But there was almost nothing more available on witchcraft.

Not witchcraft. That was not the key word. Even in the medical index, it was a man's world. Not the witches. You could not look up witches.

Satan. That was what you had to look up. That was how men labeled it. After the man. Satan. Satanic cults. Satanic rituals. Those were the key words. She punched them into the computer. And out came the list of articles.

She started with one written by Russell in 1972. Russell described a number of different levels of skepticism exemplified by various historians who had tried over the years to interpret primary sources on satanism. Therapists, it seemed, had adopted the same biases and the same forms of skepticism as historians.

A historian named Margaret Murray hypothesized that the cult of witches could be traced back to Greek and Roman worship of Artemis and Diana. One goddess with two names. An ancient cult. A cult with deep roots. That went way back. Deep roots. Basic rituals. Archetypal symbols. Jung, not Freud.

As she read on, she was able to put together a patchwork history of the Black Mass. It evolved into a parody of THE MASS. Satan as anti-Christ. Satanism as a reaction to Christianity. With the symbols. The pure symbols. The symbols of satanic ritual. The archetypal symbols. Not the theology, the basic symbols. Those were what she needed to know.

She found them. Some of them.

The number. The magic number. Thirteen. It hadn't changed in over two thousand years. Most of Chicago's high-rise apartment buildings had no thirteenth floor. The power of the number thirteen. The coven. Leslie's coven. Any coven. Then or now. That number had been etched into Leslie's memory. She hadn't just dreamed that up.

The gowns. The black gowns. The pointed hats. Witches' hats. The circle. The altar. With a naked woman on it. Flat on her back.

Women as goddesses. Not in their function as mother. Not mother goddesses. Not for reproduction. Women as priestesses. As sex goddesses. Real sex goddesses. Whore priestesses. There to fornicate in the true sense of the word. Intercourse outside of marriage.

A naked woman spread-eagled on an altar. As an altar. Totally exposed. Totally wanton. There for one purpose and one purpose only.

The chalice. The chalice of blood.

And candles. Black and white candles. Only one could be white. And they all had to be phallic. No haystacks allowed.

And a knife. To get the blood. To cut the children. But not all of the children. Not the girls.

The sacrifice. Of a child. A girl. A little girl. Not by death. By sex. A man. Men. A little girl.

By rape.

Leslie. By Kroller. That SOB!

Dennie had read enough. Who cared about the theology? That was not important. That was mere decoration. Fun. Mocking the church. Any church. It was the ritual that mattered. Thank God for therapists like John Doran who knew how to get their patients to tell their stories.

And knew enough to believe them. To believe Leslie. And help her. And understand all the destruction it had caused. The terrible damage. Right down to the core of the soul. The personality itself.

"Hi."

She all but jumped out of her chair. "Tom."

He sat down, pulled out his notebook, and started to read his notes to her. Almost as if she were a real deputy sheriff. Part of his team.

"He was signed in here as William Kroller, Jr. His therapist was a guy named Nielsen. Roger Nielsen. Apparently well-respected. Around seventy. Used to be head of the department here," he paused.

"What was the diagnosis?" she asked. Wondering if she should tell him everything she knew. That Roger Nielsen had been her sister's therapist. No, that wasn't any of his business.

"Is that important?" he asked.

"Is that important!" she exploded. "It's the whole issue."

"What are you talking about?"

Tom, she realized, could not be expected to understand what she meant, had not read what she had. He had not immersed himself in the psychiatric controversy. Nor should he have. She had to explain it to him. Where to start? The beginning. Where did it begin?

"Start at the beginning," he said.

"The beginning. That's before Rome."

"What are you talking about?"

"I need something to eat. Can we go someplace?"

They drove to a small Italian restaurant less than a mile from the medical center. On Taylor Street. In what was left of one of Chicago's oldest Italian neighborhoods. A neighborhood that had been invaded by the medical center, by public housing, and now by the new evil of gentrification. Their forebears had come here to escape the gentry. And now their children were becoming gentrified. The restaurant had all the necessary symbols. Candles in Chianti bottles.

White candles. Red checkered tablecloths. Bad friezes painted on the walls. Hanging gourds. Fake vines. The works.

And good bread. With butter, not olive oil. Neither virgin. Nor extra virgin. How could one become an extra virgin? And who would want to?

And hot minestrone, loaded with vegetables and served with fresh Parmesan cheese. The freshest. Extra fresh. Each table had its own cheese grinder. And a hunk of cheese. Grind it yourself. What could be fresher?

Their homemade pasta.

And Tom ordered a Pinot Grigio.

When they got to the cannoli—homemade, of course—and the cappuccino they both recognized that it was time to get back to work.

"I'll tell you my story," she said, "if you'll tell me yours."

He chuckled. He had a nice laugh. And a nice smile. She was such a sucker for a smile. Give her a nice smile and she'd do anything. Not quite anything.

Dennie told him everything that she'd learned about witchcraft, about satanism, about satanic ritual child abuse. She almost sounded like an expert on the subject, not a novice. She'd always been a quick learner. Then she talked about John Doran. Jungian psychology, Leslie, Leslie's father, no—her stepfather, her mother's husband, whatever, and his son, Billie Kroller. And ended with the same question. "What was Billie Kroller's diagnosis?"

Tom now understood the significance of that question. Satanic ritual abuse was a cause of multiple personality disorders. Was John Johnston a personality? Or a disguise? A nom de plume? Or whatever?

"Depression," he said.

"Just depression?"

"It's hard to say 'just depression' about somebody who just killed himself."

"You know what I mean."

He did. "Just depression. His alias was a disguise. He used that name in his life as a male. . . , " he paused.

He was so sweet, wanting to protect her from the sordid details.

"Hooker," she said.

"Yes. To keep all that hidden from his old man. Hookers almost always have . . . ah . . . stage names, so to speak."

"Tell me exactly what happened," she requested.

"He put the gun in his mouth and. . . ."

"Not the gory details."

"Okay." Most of the non-gory details were pretty straightforward. Billie had signed into the hospital the night before Doran had been killed.

But he'd kept his appointment on the next day, she reminded him. How had he managed that?

He'd had an official pass for two hours.

So he was back in the hospital by the time John Doran was killed?

Yes. All locked in according to the records.

The gun? Where had it come from?

That was a good question. The only entrance to the closed unit on Eleven Walsh had metal detectors. That meant that Billie Kroller had not brought in the gun with him.

So who had?

An orderly. In the food cart. Under a metal food warmer.

"For five hundred bucks."

"From whom?"

"Billie Kroller."

It certainly had not been a gesture.

"By the way, he couldn't have saved your life. He was signed in then, too," Tom told her.

"If he could get a gun in, he could get himself out," Dennie said speaking the thought that was on both of their minds.

Tom paid the bill and turned to her. "I've got an idea."

So did she.

"Let's go over to Doran's and find the rest of Kroller's tapes."

That had not been her idea of what to do next.

"And then we can watch them."

Nor that.

"There's only one other question," he went on. "Should we watch them at your place or mine?"

"Mine," she decided.

✳✳✳✳

A Chicago police department squad car with its lights flashing away was pulled across the entrance to the parking area in the mall in front of John Doran's office. Behind it they could see half a dozen other squad cars, all flashing away. And three, no, four fire trucks. Three pumpers, pumping away. One hook and ladder. Hooking, but not laddering.

And a veritable tumult of activity. Of men running. Shouting. Controlled chaos. Hoses. Water. Streams of water. And flames. Huge flames. A fire. More like a conflagration. Enveloping Doran's office. And all the shops near it. The video store. The dry cleaners.

Tom rolled down his window.

"You'll have to move on," the uniformed officer said.

Tom showed him his badge.

"Sorry, Lieutenant, I didn't know who you were."

"That's okay. What happened?"

"Looks like a firebomb. It was probably aimed at the video store. That one may have been a front."

"Drugs?"

"What else?"

"Professionals?"

"Yes, but sloppy ones. They missed the video store. Not by much. They hit the next storefront. Some shrink's office. Poor guy. It probably put him out of business for a while. The miss didn't matter much. Those videos are so damn flammable they caught fire, too. They burn like incendiaries."

Like incendiaries.

"All of those tapes just went poof," the officer explained.

Poof. So much for John Doran's tapes. His tapes of Billie Kroller, alias John Johnston. And of Leslie. And all of his other patients. And playmates.

Except for the four that she had.

Maybe one of those playmates had killed him. Or one of those patients. Poof. They might never know.

Even though they did not have the excuse of videotapes they needed to review, they still went back to her place, but instead of watching one of Doran's videos, they sat on her couch, almost touching as they talked. Not about the death of Billie Kroller. Or the attempt that had been made to kill her. Or how Billie Kroller had saved her life. All of that seemed to hang over them like some foreboding cloud. A subject to be avoided. Like Beth. Her whereabouts. Her activities. Her mere existence. All were equally taboo.

Tom showed her the death certificate of Jennifer Williams. She had been seven years old when she died. The cause of death was listed as severe contusions of the brain due to an automobile accident.

Not exactly surprising news. That was exactly what Kim had told her. Her little sister had died in an auto accident. That was why Kim had been so upset. The patient she had lost had been in an automobile accident. And died because of it.

"Perhaps the autopsy report will be more interesting," he said.

"Autopsy report? Did they do an autopsy on her?"

"Yes."

"Why?"

"She died suddenly. In an accident. All such sudden deaths are medical examiner's cases. There's always an autopsy. Here, look at it," he said, handing it to her.

She started to read it, not that all of it made sense to her. She understood most of the words. But not their full medical significance. Their medicolegal significance. She scanned it. Crush injury to the chest. Rib fracture. Callus formation. Healed fracture. Brain contusion. Cardiac tamponade. That was beyond her. Lacerations. Scars. Burns. Small round burns. Healed.

"Some accident," she concluded.

"Read it again."

She did. Healed fractures. Scars. Small round burns. Like burns from a cigarette. New ones. And old ones. At the same time. New fractures. And old ones. How? Why?

"It wasn't an accident."

"Bingo," he said.

"She'd been a battered kid. Battered and burned. Somebody had been beating up on Jennifer Williams. And burning her . . . and . . . who knows what else. That poor kid. And then. . . ," she halted, not certain she wanted to know.

"Somehow her father ran over her in her own driveway," Tom said.

"Oh, my God." Dennie got up and went into the bathroom and gagged. Once. Twice. Everything came up. Her entire dinner. And she kept on gagging until there was nothing left. No dinner. Just a painful emptiness. She washed her face, not bothering to replace the makeup. Who cared if her face was battered? Then she brushed her teeth and gargled with mouthwash. She felt cleaner, if not better. She negotiated her way back to the living room.

"You okay?" he asked.

"Hell, no. Are you?"

"You want me to go home?" he replied, ignoring her question.

Why couldn't men answer such simple questions? "No. I'm not ready to be that alone quite yet."

"Okay. Tell me when you are."

"I will."

"I talked to Mrs. Kroller."

Satan's concubine. The thirteenth witch.

"I asked her about the names from Leslie's list. She remembered three others for sure. The Lynns. They were neighbors. Had been for a couple of years. There was a Collins family who went to the same church. Still did. And the Bergers. She thought there was a Berger girl in kindergarten with Leslie. A fat, ugly little girl. A real beast."

"That's all she said?"

"It took an hour to get that much out of her."

"That leaves two. Two out of twelve are still unaccounted for."

"So what?" Tom mused.

"So what? What a question!"

"We know what we have to know. They all had to be people from their past whether anyone remembers the names or not."

"But they were all accomplices."

"To what? Accomplices to what?"

"Witchcraft."

"When did that become a felony?"

"Rape, then. Child abuse."

"Williams, probably. He abused his own kid. He could have done that in the privacy of his own home. Most people do it that way. With no one's help. And maybe the Felsches. But so far no one has filed any complaint."

"No complaint? What about Leslie?"

"What about her? Let's talk about Leslie. She only filed a civil suit. No criminal complaint. None at all. Why not? Could it be that she's after money, not justice?"

"Is that what you think? You cops probably think the little girls ask for it."

"Is that what you think? If it is, I'd better leave now." He got up, prepared to leave.

She reached out and grabbed his arm. "I'm sorry—it's been a long day. Please stay. And change the subject."

He didn't sit back down. Instead he crossed over to a bookshelf that was loaded with CDs and started shuffling through them.

She watched him. What would he pick? There was no Philip Glass. Something romantic, she hoped. Prokofiev's *Romeo and Juliet,* Tchaikovsky's.

He rejected all the romantics. From Berlioz to Tchaikovsky. One after the other. And finally settled on Mahler. And not the First Symphony. The Fifth. Beginning with the Funeral March.

He sat back on the couch. "I just want to say one more thing and then I'll keep my mouth shut."

Don't do that.

"Brian Havergal. Stay away from him. There, I'm done."

"I'm sorry I don't have any Philip Glass."

"How about some coffee?"

"I could make some."

"I'm not disabled," he said. "I'll make the coffee."

"Good, then I can go to the bathroom."

"You okay?"

"Yes. Are you?"

"I'll make the coffee."

Her diaphragm was where she had put it six months ago. Or had it been seven? She opened a new tube of gel. She liked doing this. It proved to her that she had made the decision. That she was in charge. It was now up to him to follow her lead. He was the one who could say no. Hold. Enough. She left off her panty hose and replaced her heavy sweater with a far lighter one. Lighter and open at the neck.

"Are you okay?" he asked.

"Why do you keep asking me that?"

"You took so long."

"It takes us longer."

"Oh," he said, as if he understood, which he clearly didn't.

He tasted so good. His mouth. His tongue. His lips felt good on her lips. On her neck. On her breasts.

And his fingers also felt good. Everywhere. She was responding. So damn quickly. Fully.

But he wasn't. Not at all. Not to her hand. Nor her tongue. Nor her mouth. Nor to anything.

He pushed her away. And then reached down and with his fingers began to massage her ever so lightly.

To penetrate her.

"My God, you're . . . you're . . . a diaphragm!"

"What did you think took so long?"

"You do want . . . to make love. To me."

"God damn right, buster. So get your act in gear." It was only when they came up for air for the second time that she added, "That's why I said my place."

Chapter
XII

Tom stayed the night. He was the first to wake up in the morning. Dennie felt him moving. She was too tired to move. And too relaxed. Where did he get all that energy?

If she wasn't so tired, maybe they could think of a good use for that energy. But she was. She watched him as he pulled on his clothes. She thought she heard him in the kitchen. She hoped he would make fresh coffee. Then he was back. He had brought her a cup. Tom put the coffee on the bedside table and kissed her gently on the forehead.

"I have to go," he said. "I have a lot of work to do." He sounded apologetic. He should.

"What time is it?" she asked.

"Six thirty."

"Why do you have to go?" Not wanting him to go. Not wanting it to end. Not wanting to be alone. Not yet.

"I still have a killer to catch."

"Not Beth."

"Of course not Beth."

She sat up in bed, exposing her naked breasts to him.

"Don't tempt me," he said.

"If I still do after last night, that's a good sign," she told him, hoping that it was.

"It's a good sign," he said.

She took a sip of her coffee. Tom had remembered. He had put just the slightest amount of milk in it. "You are a sweet man, Tom Ward."

"I'll bet you say that to all your men the morning after."

"All! What's that supposed to mean?"

"I'm sorry. I just. . . . I don't know what to say the next morning. What is the proper etiquette? I've only done this with my wife. My ex-wife, I mean. I . . . I. . . ." He was blushing. This man was actually embarrassed. They had made love and hugged and kissed and explored each other's bodies with their hands and lips and tongues and then made love again and he had no idea what to say to her the morning after and he felt embarrassed. He was sweet. And dear. And precious.

146

"I usually tell them to get lost," she said.

"What do you mean?"

"By the time I wake up and imagine them trying to grab me again, I know it was a mistake. So I can't wait to see them leave so I can wash their smell off my body and then get every last trace of them out of me. Ugh."

He stood there awkwardly. He had no idea what to say to her. This was a world that was new to him.

And she knew it.

Finally he stammered, "So what are you going to do?"

"Take a shower."

"And wash me off of you. And out. . . ."

"Not quite."

"Not quite, then what?"

She got up, stretched her arms out, giving him the most enticing view possible. "We are going to shower together and wash each other clean, a full body shower, and then you are going to put more of you in me."

"Is that a proposition?"

"It's more like an order."

"We serve and protect," he smiled at her.

"Do I need protection? I just want some service."

He never answered her question. He couldn't. She pressed her body against his, closing her mouth onto his and at the same time undoing his belt buckle.

They both already knew the answer.

✳✳✳✳

It was eleven o'clock. Tom had been gone for three hours. It was time for her to finally get up out of bed. Should she shower again? No. She enjoyed his smell. And the knowledge that part of him was still inside of her. Along with her diaphragm. Her legs felt sore. She had stretched muscles she had not stretched in months. More like eons since she had stretched them like that! If ever.

She put on her terrycloth robe, brushed her teeth, poured some more of the coffee Tom had made, put on another pot, and took the coffee into the living room to get some work done. She wanted some music. She turned on the CD player. The CD that Tom had picked the night before began spinning. Mahler. Not Mahler. And certainly not the Fifth Symphony. Nothing funereal. Nothing philosophical. Something lush. Romantic. Strauss. Richard Strauss. *Symphonia Domestica.* A tone poem of married bliss. Her half conscious choice startled her. A domestic symphony. She wasn't a domestic person. Married bliss. How could she even think of such a future?

With Tom Ward of all people. A divorced cop. He was sweet. And they were great in bed together. Not as an athletic venture. No bravura, just a combination of caring and need. Wonderfully balanced. Or had they just had a good night? Just happened to be in sync for those few hours? That she did not want to believe.

But what did she know about him? And more to the point, what did he know about her? And her sisters? They were almost like triplets. Only more so. They were her entire family. All she had in this world. Marrying one meant accepting all three of them. And he'd never even met the other two. And one he thought might well be a killer.

No. Not anymore. He didn't believe Beth had killed John Doran. He considered her to be just one of the suspects. A suspect. That meant that Tom still thought that Beth was a person who was capable of murder. That wasn't much different. And besides he was a cop. Who would want to spend a lifetime with a cop?

Beth. With Mike. Mike apparently loved Beth. Mike made her happy. Wrong. Mike made it possible for Beth to find her own happiness. That had never happened to Beth before. Would Tom make it possible for Dennie to find her own happiness?

Yes, he would. How could she know that? She wasn't sure but somehow she knew he could do that. And that she could do that for him. Like Mike and Beth. If only the world didn't get in the way.

Enough dillydallying. To work.

She sat down at her desk. There was a fax in the fax machine. It was from Mike. Speak of the devil. Bad metaphor that, all things considered. Beth hadn't called Mike last night. She'd been at Mike's the night before. But last night Mike had heard nothing. If Dennie heard from Beth, she should leave a message for Mike. At home. Mike checked the machine every hour. Not at work.

Of course, not at work. Mike was a cop. A cop who worked with Tom Ward. Dennie might not know anything about police routine or how to go about catching a killer, but she wasn't stupid.

Tom. She rubbed the sore muscles of her inner thighs. Aches and pains could be such fun. Tom.

To work. She called Sean. Had he heard from his client?

Which client?

Why was he being so devious? Then she remembered. Her line was bugged.

Could they bug faxes? What a good question. Sean ought to know the answer to that. He was into secrecy and privileged communication. She asked him.

No. That was what she needed to know. Then he started to explain the electronics of it. That she didn't need to know.

"I'll fax you," she said. And hung up. She typed out a question on her computer and faxed it to Sean Keneally.

"Have you heard from Beth?"

In three minutes she got a return fax. "Yes."

"Is she alright?"

Three minutes later another "yes" appeared.

Progress, but very slow. As frustrating as making love one stroke at a time. One insertion only. She needed a flurry. All she got was one at a time. Not Dennie's style. Her next fax contained a series of questions. Did Sean know where Beth was? Did he know how to contact her? Did he have plans to see her? To talk to her? To tell her that she was no longer the prime suspect? Could he tell her to call Dennie? There was so much she needed to tell her. Did she know about John Johnston, alias Billie Kroller? Or vice versa?

A series of answers. All of which boiled down to the fact that Sean hoped to talk to his client early that evening and that he'd relay Dennie's messages. And Sean also had a question. Tom Ward wanted to meet with him about Three Sisters Limited, not as clients but as employees. Did she mind? He could try to call it all privileged but it was a murder investigation and sometimes it was better to play along. Or at least to appear to be playing along.

She didn't mind.

Back to the phone. There were issues they could discuss openly. Had Sean talked to Leslie?

He hadn't. Why?

She was not in good shape. What an understatement. She was losing it again. John Doran had helped her. She was dependent on him and he was dead. She obviously needed a new therapist. And Dennie had promised to find her one.

"Find her one who is willing to testify," Sean advised.

"This isn't about winning a lawsuit. There are other things in this world than money."

"My mother taught me one thing. There is no situation that having more money makes worse. Especially a lot more money."

"You really are a cynic."

"Look, I want Leslie to be happy. I want her to be well. I can't make her happy. I can't make her well. Can her therapist? I sure as hell hope so. But can he guarantee it? Can you? You're goddamn right he can't. But with his help I may be able to make her rich. Will that make her happy?" He paused. The lawyer at work. On a closing argument.

"Will it make her well?" Another pause. For effect. He was good, no question about that.

"How the hell do I know? But it is the one thing I can do for her. If that's cynicism, let's make the most of it. Just make sure he'll testify."

"Leslie's new therapist could be a woman."

"Fine by me, a woman would make a great expert in this case."

"She may not want to testify."

"Try, Denise, try. Find one who will."

No sooner had she hung up than the phone rang.

"I hear you're interested in me," the deep male voice said.

"Who is this?"

"Guess."

"I'm not good at games."

"I am. Very good. Especially at one particular game. One where size really matters."

"Brian Havergal."

"Big Brian. How did you ever guess?"

"And you're good at basketball."

"My second best indoor sport," he said tantalizingly.

What a bore. Even his innuendoes were sophomoric. What could one expect from a basketball star? He was probably in sophomore classes for the second or third time. And, of course, he was into sophomore girls. Unless they were too sophisticated for him.

"And size counts in both," he continued.

What about Michael Jordan? Lots of guys were bigger. And taller. And. . . . She said nothing. This was his dime. Correction. His quarter.

"I hear you're interested in me," he repeated. Apparently he had run out of what passed for clever repartee.

"Where did you hear that?"

"Word gets around."

"What else did you hear?"

"That you have good legs." Matter of factly. Not as a compliment. As a statement of fact. As if she had fulfilled a necessary prerequisite. And perhaps she had.

"I'm free tonight," he said. "About seven."

"I'm not."

"I don't like no's."

"That's what I heard," she informed him. "That you don't take no for an answer."

"I don't know what you're talking about."

"Oh, I suppose no girl ever said no to you."

"You've got that right. Not to Big Brian."

"Well, this one has."

"Has what?"

"Said no." She hung up. Asshole! Could Big Brian have killed someone? Could he have killed John Doran? It seemed unlikely. But maybe it wasn't. Brian was supposed to be an NBA first-round pick. What was that worth? Ten million. Twenty. Who knew these days? Not her. And there was no situation that more money made worse.

Not true.

Money. Possible money. Future money. Money that needed to be protected. There was a motive. A real motive. Not just for whodunits. For the real work-a-day world of butcher knives in the back. Not a theological concept. Not saying the Mass backwards or whatever. Not witchcraft.

Money.

And he didn't even have to do it himself. He could have hired someone. One of the hookers. That girl. She'd do anything for money. For enough money. Even murder?

Or had that hooker just set Doran up? Nice ambiguity there. Someone could have hired one of his hookers to give him more than he had bargained for. Or to set him up for the kill. All she had to do was to strip. Tell her story with a few gestures. Be as enticing as she could.

Bump and grind. Naked. With touching. Of herself. And then him. That was what hookers did. Or at least that was what Dennie thought they did.

John Doran. The naked therapist. Naked. Vulnerable. And bingo. Slip a knife into his rib cage. It had to be an easier way to make a living than giving blow jobs to strangers. If she had to pick one, she knew which one she'd pick. But that was why she hadn't slept with a man in over six months. How many of her friends could make that statement? Not enough of them.

But then they'd have to kill the girl, too. The girl who had told Brian's story to John Doran. The girl who had been raped by Brian. What was her name? R. It began with an R. R something. Robin. Robin Riegel.

Tom. She called Tom. He was out. She left a message. She needed to talk to him. And she did. Among other things.

She had, she realized, become the very model of a modern private detective. Not pounding the pavement. Not a flat foot. Not a gumshoe. But working the phone. A flat ear.

Or a flat ass.

Would Tom like it that way? Did he really care? Or did he tell that to all the girls? My first time since. . . . It was a good line. It worked. It made her feel special. Very special.

He hadn't made love like a first-timer. Someone who hadn't made love in four years. Did that make him a virgin again? Had she deflowered him? She hoped so. Or. . . .

She stood up. The Strauss was over. She needed something peppier. With driving rhythms. Stravinsky. *Rite of Spring.* Complete with a virgin sacrifice. And as it played, she began to exercise. In rhythm with the music. With one of its rhythms. The phone interrupted her. And none too soon. It was Tom.

"You left a message."

"Darling," she said, "I miss you."

"This is official police business."

On a bugged line, she remembered.

"Robin," she explained. "Robin Riegel. The girl Big Brian raped."

"Allegedly raped."

"Raped."

"Twice on the same night. In her apartment."

"She was raped," Dennie insisted.

"You sound convinced."

"I am. Is she okay?"

"I have no idea," Tom replied. "Why are you asking?"

She explained her theory. Even to her it sounded flimsy. But it was a possibility. Someone could have sent in one of those hookers to do it. Or to set him up. It had to be easier to kill a guy than spend a lifetime giving sex to strangers.

Fortunately, most women didn't think that way.

Fortunately! He went around getting sex from strangers.

Absolutely not. But if women thought like she did, there would be more such murders. And he'd be in Vice. He hated Vice. What should he do?

Make certain that Robin Riegel was okay.

He'd check on her.

And she should stay far away from him?

"From whom?" innocently.

"Havergal."

"Why?"

"He raped that girl."

"You didn't sound that convinced before," she said.

"You know what I mean."

"It all depends on whose girl got raped. Or might get raped."

"Maybe."

"If he were charged with rape, what would happen?" she asked.

"We'd have to arrest him."

"No, to his career?"

"Nobody would touch him. The Bulls once drafted a guy about ten years ago. Hailey. Or Bailey. I think. Somebody Bailey. He'd been charged with rape in a dorm and acquitted. And he was hounded to death. All over the league. Protesters. Mobs. And that was a decade ago. When date rape. . . ."

"Wasn't really a crime yet."

"Yeah."

"That could cost Brian millions," she said.

"Yep. No one would touch him with a ten-foot pole."

"I think that's what he wants to do to me."

"What? Oh. That's not a joke."

"I'm not laughing."

"Be careful," he reiterated. "And don't change your views on sex. I'd rather have you kill somebody."

"See you around, Lieutenant."

She looked up a number and placed yet another call. After replacing Stravinsky with Bruckner. No more virginal sacrifices. The virgins of this world had sacrificed far too much. Before, during, and after.

She told Dr. Nielsen's receptionist that her name was Cater and that she needed to talk to the doctor and then she waited.

"Elizabeth," the voice said. "How are you?"

"This is her sister."

"Jessica?"

"Dennie. Denise."

"We've never met."

"I know. I was away then."

"How is your sister?"

"Fine. She's doing well. Thanks to your help."

"She's a fine young woman. I hope I helped her help herself."

"That's what I called to talk about. Helping one of your patients."

"I can't really discuss one of my patients with you. It's what's called privileged communication."

"I understand all about that. I wanted to talk to you about a different patient of yours, John Johnston."

"Who?"

"Bill Kroller. Billie."

Once again the physician was hesitant. He couldn't talk about a patient. Even a dead patient. The patient's rights had to be protected. Even after death.

"Can you answer some general questions?"

How general?

Diagnosis. Differential diagnosis. About the nature of the diagnostic process. About childhood abuse. About rituals.

In general, he could, but why did she need the information?

She summarized her needs. And her role. She told him about Leslie and John Doran's treatment of Leslie.

"All that witchcraft rigamarole, I suspect," was his reply.

She told him about John Doran's murder. That did impress him. Did he know that Billie Kroller was also seeing John Doran? He didn't. Or about his activities as a male prostitute. His what? She explained. No. But he'd only been his patient for a couple of days.

Didn't that mean that Bill Kroller had two identities? Two separate lives.

No, it didn't. Such cases were rare. Patients often consciously invented second personalities but true multiple personalities were rare. They were called dissociative states. Quite rare. Some analysts doubted they even existed. He didn't, but they were exceptionally rare.

But what about satanic rituals?

The professional literature on the topic of satanic ritual abuse is nearly nonexistent.

She knew that. But there were adult survivors who described experiences of satanic ritual abuse during childhood. There were reports in which children described the chanting or singing. And all of those symbols. The witches' costumes, masks, candles, and the drinking of blood. And human sacrifice. Like *Rite of Spring,* she thought to herself. Without Stravinsky. Or Nijinsky.

He'd read some such reports.

So had she. And she believed them.

He didn't. They were the patients' own distortions. Their own fantasies.

How could that be?

They often were hypnotized.

So what? Hypnotism freed the mind, the memory.

But, he countered authoritatively, memories elicited under hypnosis were notably unreliable.

She didn't know that.

He did. Remarkably unreliable. Real recollections and fantasies were equally vivid. Equally well remembered. Equally intense. And equally believable or unbelievable, he concluded.

What was his diagnosis? On Billie Kroller.

"Depression."

"Simple depression."

"Is depression ever simple?"

"No," she conceded. Never that simple.

"Mr. Kroller didn't have multiple personalities. He was one person. He liked to try to escape but consciously. Like a child playing a game."

She thanked him.

For what?

For helping Beth.

"Give her my regards. She is a fine young woman. I hope to dance at her wedding someday."

What a nice man. "So do I. Wait. I have one more question. If it's all just fantasy, why do so many of them dream the same sort of dreams. Witches. Circles. Altars. Candles."

"Do they?"

"Yes."

"I don't know."

"Maybe Jung was right," she suggested.

"I wouldn't bet on that, Ms. Cater," rejecting her blasphemy.

She might have to.

"Take care of yourself."

"I will," she reassured him. Had that been politeness or something else? Some sort of warning. A reminder that she needed to take care of herself? "You too," she replied. Politeness? Or a word of caution?

She wasn't sure. She did know she had more work to do. She called Slatter's office. She would like to talk to him again. He would be free at three. That was perfect. She had time for lunch and a shower.

✳✳✳✳

She drove to the Jung Institute. A cab would have been cheaper, but she liked the 'vette. It was far slower and so much less convenient. But the last time she'd waited for a cab hadn't been fun. And Billie Kroller wouldn't be around to protect her. Was Beth? She sure hoped so.

It wasn't until she pulled into the parking lot that she was sure that a car had been following her. Probably not a 'vette enthusiast. It was a different car than before. With a driver wearing sunglasses. It was bright and sunny, but not that bright. Nor that sunny. It had to be Beth. Thank God. Beth. Alive. Well. And protecting her.

Slatter was as affable as ever. Had she found a therapist?

She hadn't. What she needed was an expert on witchcraft.

Why?

To testify about witchcraft. She explained the nature of her need. Then they talked about the ritual. And all the symbols. Why were people so skeptical?

Who in particular?

Nielsen. Roger Nielsen.

Pompous Freudian.

Was that the reason? Doctrinal debate?

What else? Then Slatter asked her the same question that she had asked Nielsen in almost the exact same words. If it was all just fantasy, why did so many of them dream the same dream? With the same symbols?

"Because it's true," she suggested.

"Yes."

Would he help Leslie as an expert? Not on Leslie. On the whole process.

He would.

About satanic cults as a cause of psychiatric distress?

He would. Such abuse caused serious behavioral problems. Depression. And multiple personalities.

In the same family, could one abused child become depressed and another have multiple personalities?

Not only could. Did. Very commonly.

She told him about Leslie. And her half brother. They had such different problems. Could they both be caused by the same trauma? By satanic ritual abuse? She was proud of herself—she'd used the correct terminology.

Yes. What were his problems?

It was strange. Nielsen couldn't talk about his patient but Slatter could. After all, Billie wasn't Slatter's patient. Medical ethics. They didn't apply to her. Any more than that restraining order had. She told him all about Bill Kroller alias John Johnston.

It was, he was certain, a classic case of multiple personalities caused by satanic ritual abuse.

Why hadn't Nielsen realized that?

Doctors only heard what they wanted to hear.

BINGO.

❋❋❋❋

Someone was following her car. Who? She couldn't tell. The same person? No. It wasn't even the same car. A man. It was a man. Big. But white. A goon? A white goon? Not all goons were black. Probably not even most of them. Probably not even most of Kroller's goons. Then the car was gone. She'd probably been wrong. Paranoid. No one was following her. Not Beth. Not some white goon. No one.

Where should she go?

Home. It was warm and sunny for February. She'd go jogging. In the park. She gave the 'vette to A.C. but kept the keys. She might need it later. A quick change and she was out in the park. It felt good. Perfect running weather. Cold but sunny. And dry. Perfect for a jog in the park. In the empty park. Almost empty. Someone else was jogging. On a day like this there should have been a lot of other joggers. There weren't. Just one man.

Behind her.

One man.

One big man.

A mountain of a man.

Behind her.

Fifty yards behind her.

She picked up her pace.

So did he.

Faster yet.

So did he.

Her heart was pounding. She never was good at running. Beth was the athlete. Dennie knew that she couldn't keep this up for long. She looked over her shoulder.

He didn't look winded at all. He smiled at her. God, he was enormous. And smiling. The bastard!

And waving at her. And picking up his pace.

She looked around. She was all alone. In the middle of the park. Her only hope was to get out of the park. And fast. She could not go any faster.

He could.

Only twenty yards separated them now.

There was still no one in sight. Except for one man. One goon. One big white goon. Someone had been following her. It hadn't been paranoia. Her heart was pounding harder. And faster. And her head was beginning to throb. And pound. Not the spinning again. Please God.

Shit! He was only ten yards away.

Five yards.

The pounding was not going away. It was changing. Into a state of total panic.

Three.

None.

He tackled her. She fell to the ground with him on top of her, pressing her to the ground. Underneath him.

She waited for the blow.

Or the gun shot.

Or the knife blade. The blade of a butcher knife.

Or a muffler around her neck.

This was how her life was going to end. Not a bang. Not a whimper. Just an ending.

She felt him shift his weight. He was astride her now, his knees resting on the ground on either side of her. He grabbed her shoulder and started to roll her over underneath him. He was going to look at her before he killed her.

And she at him.

She tried to resist.

He yanked harder. And her body had no choice. She was flat on her back and he was astride her, looking down, smirking, getting ready to kill her. She was frightened. Petrified. Immobile. Almost frozen by her own terror.

Panic.

Pounding in her chest and head.

Beth, save me.

Beth!

Tom.

Tom.

Someone.

Anyone.

No.

He wasn't going to kill her.

He was going to rape her.

He was merely going to rape her.

"No one ever says no to me."

It was Brian Havergal. Not one of Kroller's goons. Brian Havergal. Big Brian. And he wasn't going to kill her. He was only going to fuck her. To rape her.

Thank God.

Thank God?

A simple rape.

She felt her terror begin to evaporate. And her fear. And her immobility.

He was pulling on her sweat pants. Trying to pull them down.

She started to move, to resist. To squirm. To fight.

"I like a little spirit," he said.

"I don't."

They weren't alone. There was a car next to them. It was the car she'd seen following her before. Earlier. On her way to Slatter's office. And there was also a driver. Getting out of the car. A driver wearing sunglasses.

And a badge.

And a gun. A great big gun. Bigger than Brian's. She was sure of that.

Mike.

Dennie had never been so happy to see anyone.

"Son, I think you'd better get the fuck out of here."

"I. . . ."

"Do you know this man?" Mike asked.

By now Brian was off of her and she had struggled to her feet.

"Yes. His name is Brian Havergal. And he wanted to rape me."

"We were just playing."

"Did he take his prick out?"

"No."

"No rape attempt, legally speaking. But I tell you, young man, if I ever see you trying this again, I'll shoot it off."

Dennie laughed.

"Bitch," Brian spat out at them.

"He's done it before," she said.

"He has?"

"Bullshit!"

"To Robin Riegel."

"That whore. She was begging for it. Well, she got it and now she's complaining. She even told her fuckin' shrink. Well, he. . . ."

"He what?" Dennie asked. Perhaps this man could have killed Doran. Or had him killed.

"Nothing. Nothing at all."

"Shall I shoot him now?" Mike asked, waving the gun and then pointing it at Brian's genitals.

"Naw. Let him go," she said.

"Run along, boy," Mike said, pointing all the time.

Brian did. Faster than he had caught up with Dennie.

"Mike, why are you here?"

"Tom Ward assigned me to look after you. He's my boss."

"He's a sweet man."

"Not my type," Mike chuckled.

Dennie laughed. She was alive and in love. My God, she was. Both.

Chapter
XIII

Mike made the coffee for them. It was very strong. The aroma smelled quite good to Dennie. Like an old friend. Mike gave her a cup without putting any milk in it.

"I take milk in mine," Dennie said, getting up from the couch. She could get her own. This was her apartment.

"Beth doesn't."

The forbidden name had been spoken. "I know. She's my sister."

Dennie went into her kitchen and brought the milk back with her and poured a small amount into her coffee.

Then it all spilled out of Mike. Mike and Beth were not ones to spill their guts easily. But something different was going on now. They'd had their problems over the three years they'd been together. The good times and the bad. They'd broken up and come back together half a dozen times. But no matter how bad it got, how angry either of them became, they both knew that they would come back together. And they always had. Time and time again.

"I'm worried. I might lose her," Mike said. "And I do love her. And I . . . I . . . think she loves me."

"She does," Dennie reassured Mike. "Beth does love you."

"Then why am I feeling drained of that love? Threatened with its loss? That this had been some sort of a fond farewell. Almost like a wake."

That was not a question Dennie could answer. Maybe it was one of Newton's laws. Conservation of love. There could only be so much love in anyone's family. So as her love for Tom grew, that love had to come from somewhere. So Beth's had to become less. What a silly notion. This was love, not physics. And Newton was wrong. This was the age of Einstein. Of non-Newtonian physics, whatever that meant. Love, like energy, could be created. New love. Her love for Tom. She was happy that Mike was in love. Was Tom? Was she? In the way that Mike and Beth were? A love that rode out the storms. That survived the problems of living.

Dennie and Mike had never talked before. It was so reassuring to hear what Mike said about Beth. To feel Mike's emotion. To realize the depth of Mike's love. To know that Beth had not just found a lover but someone to have and to love her. Had she? And the nagging undercurrent. Why was Beth willing to give up all of this? Was she willing to? Why did Mike feel an impending loss. A virtual desertion.

To someone else?

Of course not. That had happened once and Beth had come running back. It wasn't someone else. There wasn't any third party. There had to be some other reason.

What could it be?

Had she. . . ? No, Dennie refused to believe that.

Mike told her every detail of their lives. How they had met. How they had become lovers. What they meant to each other.

Would Tom someday be able to sit down with Beth and tell her all of that? Would she?

The phone rang. Twice. It was Tom Ward. He was downstairs. In the lobby. As soon as she pushed the buzzer he'd be on his way up. She pushed it. And sat down on the couch. Mike let him in.

"I hear that Sergeant O'Rourke here saved your life."

"More like my ass," she said.

Tom turned to the other officer and said, "And for that I thank you, Michelle. It's an ass well worth saving."

Dennie was glad he felt that way.

"Do you two know each other?" Tom continued.

"Mike is Beth's lover," Dennie said matter-of-factly. A fact. Not a revelation.

To Tom this was more like a revelation than a piece of good news. "Sergeant O'Rourke, you knew I was looking for her."

"I know, Tom, but . . . my God, she didn't kill anyone."

"I know that, but I needed to talk to her. I still do."

Chapter
XIV

It was hard to tell which of them was the most upset. They seemed to take turns pacing back and forth across Dennie's living room. First Tom, then Mike, then Dennie herself. There was a continuing bustle of activity, none of which produced any meaningful result. More like Brownian motion than real activity. Pacing. Changing seats. Staring at one picture. Then another. Putting on a CD. Taking it off. Turning the CD player off. Turning it back on. Fumbling with the books on the bookshelves. The videotapes. Wandering into other rooms. Into the kitchen. Making coffee. Returning with the coffeepot. Offering the others more. Turning it down. Offering cold drinks. Turning them down. Wine. Something to eat. Some pop. And changing the subject. Insistently. Unendingly. Always changing the subject. But continuing to talk. A true Brownian conversation. But always returning to the same subjects. Over and over again

Where was Beth? None of them knew. Who had seen her last? Mike. She told them that a dozen times at least. When? Two nights before. Beth had been at Mike's that night.

Had Beth said anything about John Doran? About his murder? About what she had seen? Whom she had seen? Beth had been outside Doran's office that night watching. She was there to get something on Doran, something that Sean Keneally could have used to convince Doran to testify as an expert witness for Leslie.

"No," Mike said over and then over again. To each of their questions. "Mostly we talked about us." That was usually enough for Beth. She was usually so reticent. That night she hadn't been. And she was sweeter. More gentle. She was actually sad. "Not sad to be with me. More like sorrowful. It was almost as if she were saying goodbye to me. Nostalgic. I didn't know."

It was time for Dennie to make a confession. She became the one who was pacing.

"A confession?" Tom inquired. Certainly not innocently. He was a cop, not a priest. To him confession translated into guilt. Not sin, but crime. "Of what?"

Dennie hesitated. This was not going to be easy. Falling into bed was easy. Pleasing a man was easy. Coming clean with a man you might really love wasn't easy. Was she in love? What else could make it this difficult. She walked over to the CD. It was time for a change. Off with the CD player. On with the TV set. Then on with the VCR. Now all she needed was a tape. And she knew which one. She plucked it off her shelf. The videotape of the three sisters' family vacation. Patty, Maxine, and Laverne at play. More like Larry, Curly, and Mo.

Tom had no interest in a family vacation video, he complained. Was she going to show him the other men in her past life?

"Give it a chance, our family will grow on you."

The screen lit up. And on it they could see an image. Fuzzy at first. Then clearly.

The image on her TV screen was that of a man's backside. The man was completely naked. The camera seemed to be focused on the lower part of his spine. About four inches above the crease of his buttocks. And about six inches below the handle of a knife. It was a wooden handle of a butcher knife and the knife was sticking out of his back. Out of the left side of his back, just to the left of his spine and just above his rib cage. It had definitely entered his chest. Blood had collected at the base of the knife. . . . Not much blood.

The man was not moving. Nor was the camera. And there was noise.

"Damn," said Mike.

"Doran! That's Doran's dead body. And not too dead. I mean not dead for too long," said Tom. "Where did you get this?"

"From Beth," Dennie told them. That was part of her confession. Baring her soul.

"When?" Tom asked. "Exactly when?"

"The morning after."

The full meaning of that took a moment to set in.

"Hi," Beth's voice said. "I'm back. I was just putting a fresh tape in Doran's setup. In case you didn't recognize him. That's Doran. John Doran. Not exactly his best side. Just his most appropriate. His camera is fixed in the ceiling. The actual recording goes on in a little alcove behind his desk."

The scene never changed.

"The camera never moves. It just focuses on his couch," the voice said coldly. "He was dead when I got here. I didn't kill him. But it sure looks like he was killed by a left-handed woman while they were making love."

"It sure does, at that," Mike said.

"Mike would kill me."

"Damn right," Mike agreed. Almost a participant.

They watched the entire tape. Transfixed by a single indelible image and a halting narration.

"I'll be okay. I won't be home for a while. So I'd appreciate it if you could call Mike for me. At home. Tell Mike not to worry. Mike is such a worrywart. Like a little old lady. Not a big strong cop."

The tape was over. Beth's voice stopped. Dennie turned off the TV. Tom demanded to know if she was withholding any other evidence.

No, she wasn't.

Tom needed to talk to her sister. More than ever. Beth was a witness. A key witness. Perhaps the most important witness of all. She was the first person to see John Doran dead. That might not be quite as good as the last person to see him alive but Tom had to talk to her, to interview her.

Mike said she'd tell Beth when she saw her again. If. If she saw her again. Dennie tried to reassure her. It wasn't easy. Tom repeated his official request to Dennie. She would relay the same message. If and when. When and if.

That was not good enough for Tom. He would also tell Sean Keneally. If Beth didn't come in on her own he'd have to have a subpoena issued. A warrant.

Mike understood. She was a cop.

So did Dennie and she wasn't. It was time for a change. Time for a brand-new question. Who were the other suspects? Who had killed John Doran?

Mike said nothing. Nor did Tom. Were the two of them playing at being cops? And she was the outsider to be kept in the dark. It was okay to sleep with her, but this was official business.

"Havergal," Dennie suggested to get the conversation on track.

"Why?" Mike asked. "What would have been his motive?"

"Money. An NBA contract," Dennie said, trying to sound knowledgeable.

"What's this got to do with some NBA contract?" Mike asked.

Dennie explained as well as any professional sportswriter could have.

"Is he that good?" Mike asked her, while Tom listened. Was this just routine? Good cop-bad cop. Inquisitive cop-silent cop. She liked the silent one.

"I don't know. According to the Chicago papers he's an All-American." That was all she knew about him, what she had read in the newspapers. Not very reliable sources.

Tom was skeptical. Not mute, thank God, but very skeptical.

"Why should he kill Doran? Brian didn't rape Doran. Doran wasn't even there."

"Doran made the charge real. He gave it credibility. Look, Robin was just a girl he screwed and then jilted. That would be Brian's story. That she was a basketball groupie. Willing to spread her legs for any guy who could put the ball in the hoop. And look, had she been beaten up? Hell, no. Was she injured? Negative. Had she called the cops? Gone to her ob-gyn? No. So she must have wanted it. All sour grapes. No big deal. Girls beg for it and then cry foul all the time. It's part of the game if you're a big star. But she did do something. She went to see John Doran."

"Why was that so important?" Mike asked. He was a dogged inquisitor.

Because Doran was a psychotherapist and he was treating a patient for date rape. That would give her story credence. Validity. And in a civil suit, it would go to prove damages.

"Perhaps," Tom said, sounding a bit less skeptical. "But did Havergal know that Doran knew about the date rape?"

"He did. He told us that much," Dennie told him. "And he didn't know that Doran wouldn't testify."

Brian might be a suspect, grudgingly. "But Doran's testimony wouldn't stand up in a court of law."

It might not be the court of law that mattered here. It was a higher court. Public opinion might be what counted.

"Havergal," Tom conceded. He was finally willing to take him seriously as a potential suspect.

Then there were the Krollers, singly or as a pair. In any order.

Didn't they know that Doran wouldn't testify? That he hated to go to court. No. Dennie didn't think so. Doran was listed as an expert witness.

Had Doran ever given his deposition?

Not yet. So what could they do? Simple. Get rid of him. And all of his tapes. And what did Leslie have left as a case?

Not much, Tom agreed.

All that Leslie had, Dennie summarized, were twelve names. Which she didn't remember very well. And some of which she didn't even recognize.

"Not exactly a sure winner," Mike editorialized.

"And two abused kids," Dennie added. "Don't forget the abused kids. Both of whom are dead."

And therefore unable to testify. All that certainly left the Krollers, loving parents of Leslie and the late Billie Kroller, on their short list.

Could Billie have killed Doran?

He could. He could have gotten out of that not so locked unit, killed him, and then gotten back in. But even if he had, he couldn't have burned down the office.

They had a fourth candidate. Their list was growing. Was there a fifth? Arson wasn't the issue. Murder was.

"Leslie," Dennie said.

"You don't think she did it?" Tom said.

"Of course not. I was just thinking about her. And what to do for her. She needs a new therapist."

Who?

Dennie had an idea. Roger Nielsen, maybe. Dennie had faith in him. And he'd helped Beth so. And he was a skeptic.

Meaning?

He didn't believe in witches. In satanic ritual cults. So that when Leslie convinced him, he'd testify for her. He has great credentials. He'd make a great expert witness.

It was almost seven. They were all exhausted. Mike was going to go home in case Beth called. Or came by. Tom had a meeting with Sean Keneally. And Dennie was going to go to bed.

Alone.

She was too tired for anything else. Tom said he would call her in the morning. He didn't seem disappointed enough. They could have just held each other. He certainly hadn't argued very much. Men!

✳✳✳✳

Beth did see Mike that night. They made love but hardly talked at all. Mike was all talked out. And Beth was once again her reticent self. And she refused to stay the night. Mike relayed the message. She was a cop in real life. Beth was willing to talk to Tom Ward. Her lawyer could set it up.

When she said goodbye, Mike somehow knew it was a final goodbye.

But she did not know why.

✳✳✳✳

There was a fax waiting for Dennie when she got to her desk at seven thirty. It had arrived even earlier that morning. And it wasn't from Beth. Or Sean. Or even Tom.

The fax was from Roger Nielsen. It was a copy of an article from some medical journal named *Dissociation.* Whatever that meant.

Wait, she knew what that meant. People, patients who dissociated, dis-associated part of themselves. Who distanced themselves from some part of themselves. That was dissociation. All that psych did serve a purpose after all. The patients dissociated themselves from their feelings or from an urge. Or an emotion. Or a thought pattern. From an unacceptable emotion. Or belief. Or a second personality. Like people who had multiple personalities. Like Billie Kroller.

The article was by two psychotherapists named Coons and Grier. One was an M.D. One wasn't. Grier was a Ph.D. They were both from Indianapolis. The Indiana University School of Medicine. Professors of psychiatry. They had all the right credentials. The article was entitled "Factitious disorder (Munchausen type) involving allegations of ritual satanic abuse: a case report."

What a title. A title that said it all. If you understood the words. And Dennie thought that she did. She knew what factitious disorder meant. A fancy phrase meaning fake disease. No disease at all. Factitious, artificial, a pack of lies. That was what Baron Munchausen had done. Made up stories. Told lies. About himself. That was what Munchausen type meant. Munchausen syndrome. A patient who made up his own diseases. His own disorder. His medical history. Or hers. And went from hospital to hospital, from doctor to doctor, convincing them that he was sick. That she was sick. One or the other.

And the key phrase. The mother of all phrases. *Ritual satanic abuse.* Allegations of ritual satanic abuse. Allegations! A rather pejorative term, that.

It was the case report of a 25-year-old woman who had been hospitalized after threatening suicide. She had alleged that she had been the victim of ritual satanic abuse. A careful evaluation including history taking, clinical observation, request for collateral information, and psychological testing not only failed to corroborate her story, but pointed instead to a diagnosis of factitious disorder of the Munchausen type.

It was certainly clear why Roger Nielsen had sent this article to her. Nielsen was clearly beyond mere skepticism.

The article began with a brief review of the present state of knowledge, starting with the fact that ritual abuse involving satanic cults had recently been linked to dissociative disorders. Not a revolutionary concept to Dennie.

Dissociative states. That meant multiple personalities. The Billie Krollers of this world. But one of the problems with nearly all of the recent case reports of satanic abuse was the lack of independent corroboration.

That was what Sean had said. That was why he'd hired them. To investigate the coven of witches. Find those other witches. The accomplices. And the other victims. Like Happy Felsch. And Kim's little sister. Two more victims. What more collaboration did you need?

According to Coons and Grier such collaboration was very important because some of the patients' accounts of satanic abuse strained credibility. Strained credibility! Whose? Not hers. Not Happy Felsch's. That was for damn sure. The nerve of these experts. These so-called experts.

The woman had been hospitalized in a community mental health center after making a dramatic suicide attempt. She told them that she had escaped from a satanic cult several months previously and that ever since then she had gone from one women's shelter to another through a series of "underground safe houses" in a transcontinental flight to freedom. A modern version of the underground railway. From a different sort of slavery. White, not black. She also told them she had been the victim of ritual physical and sexual abuse by her father and other cult members. She had witnessed animal sacrifice and the ritual killing of her mother. She had been forced to act as a "breeder" of babies used for sacrifice. Ripped untimely from her womb as part of the ritual.

It was all there. Just as it had been described in Roman times. The same satanic ritual. Unchanged after all these centuries. Why hadn't they believed her? Such things happened. They had been happening for years. Decades. Centuries. Millennia. Since the dawn of time.

At the time of her admission the patient had been living with a Christian "foster family" for about a month. Immediately after a ritual exorcism she became "deaf" and attempted to kill herself.

Right out of *The Exorcist*. But no pea soup. Just satanic terror. Belief in the devil didn't matter. It was the cult. The ritual. The process, which destroyed its victims.

Early in the course of her hospitalization the patient was mute. She claimed amnesia for the last two years of her life, although she was able to write a voluminously detailed account of her abuse during her first twenty-three years. She told about fifteen to twenty pregnancies with over two-thirds ending as ritual abortions. The poor girl!

She wrote that she was having flashbacks of previous abuse. A preliminary diagnosis of post-traumatic stress disorder was made. Because of her amnesia and regressive, almost child-like behavior, a diagnosis of multiple personality disorder was also considered. How generous of them! But no attempt at all had ever been made to collect collateral information or to administer psychological testing during this hospitalization. Treatment, both psychological and psychopharmacological, was begun

Numerous lengthy treatment sessions were held. They did not help. At the end of her three-week hospitalization, she was committed to a tertiary care treatment facility. At that time her psychiatrist, the psychologists, her primary therapist, the nursing personnel, and the "foster family" all firmly believed that she had been a bona fide victim of a satanic cult. Good for them.

They finally pieced her true story together from old records. It was a story of lying, stealing, and runaway behavior during her preteen years. Unproven accusations of paternal incest at age fifteen. Leaving school in the eleventh grade. She probably withdrew long before he did. The accusations of incest began in the late 1970s, when incest had become a popular topic. Give her a break. Incest didn't start in the seventies. She produced two children out of wedlock and both were removed to foster care. By age twenty-five she had been hospitalized at least ten times in five states and had a lengthy criminal record including theft, making false accusations of rape, and threatening the foster parents of one of her children. She worked off and on. Her most recent flight began when she broke up with a boyfriend. Her mother was alive but she had been abandoned by her husband. The stories of satanic abuse did not begin until after she had observed the Geraldo Rivera television special on satanism.

Score one for Geraldo. He at least believed these abused women.

After one month of hospitalization and just prior to the initial receipt of her old records, she escaped from the hospital. Since then she had been lost to follow-up.

The authors then interpreted the case. They admitted that extreme abuse by satanic cult members might exist but the clinical picture in their case was more compatible with a diagnosis of factitious disorder. She had repeatedly changed her story to fit known data. But there were always inconsistencies in her history, numerous hospitalizations in many states, refusal to cooperate with the evaluation, extensive knowledge of hospital routine, lack of observable symptomatology, extreme disdain for treatment personnel, and rapid disappearance once her real history had become obvious. This patient met the criteria for Munchausen syndrome, but with a psychiatric presentation as first reported in 1977 by Gelenberg. Another article to peruse.

Coons and Grier were so damn smug. SOBs. Advising others to assume that the women were lying. Abused women. Sexually abused. Raped. She was angry now. If she could only convince Nielsen. And these two jerks from Indiana.

She called Roger Nielsen. She wanted him to interview a patient.

That was possible. What was the problem?

She explained. In detail. Leaving out only the issue of his becoming an expert witness. That could come later. First Leslie had to convince him. Convert him.

The name Leslie English meant nothing to him. That was strange. He'd been treating her almost-brother. She said nothing.

How about nine tomorrow morning?

She'd make sure Leslie got there. Where should they go?

Eleven Walsh. One of the treatment rooms. She could observe. He was going to invite a couple of other people also. Kris Swensen.

Another skeptic to be converted. Dennie liked that. Did he know Dr. Coons? Or Dr. Grier? From Indianapolis.

He didn't know them personally.

Too bad. If he had, he could have invited them. He declined. Dr. Nielsen wanted Dennie to explain the procedure to her friend. And be in the room by nine.

That would not be a problem.

And it wasn't. Once she'd explained it carefully to Leslie. Leslie did need an expert witness to testify on her behalf. And she knew her story was the truth. All she had to do was to tell the truth. If Roger Nielsen was as good as Dennie said, he'd recognize the truth of her story.

"He is," Dennie reassured her.

Leslie would be there. They'd meet at eight forty-five in the lobby of the Walsh building.

✳✳✳✳

Dennie had been out of bed for only two hours and she was already tired, but she had more work to do. She'd take a break. A shower. Some exercise. Breakfast. A call to Tom Ward. He was out. She left a message. A call to Mike. She was also out. Dennie left another message.

Back to work. She called the Department of Neurology at Austin Flint. And finally got through to Dr. Swensen. After the two women introduced themselves, Kris took the lead. "Paul told me about your interest in witchcraft. And I just got a call from Roger Nielsen."

Kris was going to help him design the interview and she was going to be behind that greenish mirror. How could she help Dennie?

Dennie wanted to know what to listen for. What were the symbols of true ritual satanic cults?

Kris helped her construct a list. Witches. Thirteen of them. Dressed in black. Wearing gowns. And hats. Witches' hats. These hats were an important symbol.

And the dancing. In a circle. Around an altar. With some sort of fire. Most often a big bonfire. And candles. Black and white candles. But only one white one.

With a woman on the altar. Naked. Exposed. To be violated.

How?

As many ways as possible. First with objects. Like the candles. Then by men. Men dressed as goats.

Then came the good part.

The good part?

The ritual sacrifice. Of a fetus. Or a child. Usually a fetus, ripped out of a woman.

What about saying the Mass? Backwards.

Only in Catholic countries. That was not needed. And not a primary symbol.

What about the spilling of the semen and then consuming it? And the blood?

Kris had forgotten the blood. That usually came earlier.

When?

Before the violation. Blood. In the chalice, of course. That was everything.

That was more than enough.

Kris would see Dennie at nine then. It ought to be fun.

Fun!

Dennie called Sean and told him the plan. He approved. He might try to be there. He'd also tell the Krollers' lawyer. He didn't want them to try to bar Roger Nielsen as an expert witness at some later time.

Could they demand to be there?

Yes.

But Leslie wouldn't want them there.

They could demand whatever they wanted, but they had no legal right to be there. Neither the lawyers nor the Krollers themselves. He'd make that crystal clear. And so would the judge.

Dennie felt relieved.

Had Sean seen Tom?

He had. He'd let Tom tell her about it. He had a client waiting for him.

Dennie felt like running in the park until she recalled her last run. And the urge left her.

Was Havergal really an NBA prospect? She had no way to judge that, but she knew who did. That writer who was a friend of Beth's. He was a real sports nut. He'd written that book about black baseball stars. Bingo something. And Johnny Bench's autobiography.

What was his name? Brashler. Bill Brashler. His number was in her card file. She called him. His voice was deep, resonant, sexy. He'd make a great announcer. She introduced herself as Beth Cater's sister.

He remembered Beth. She'd taken a writing course with him. How was she?

"Fine." Did he follow basketball? College basketball? DePaul?

His neighborhood team, so to speak.

She had a question, about Brian. Big Brian Havergal.

"Fire away."

"Is he an NBA prospect?"

"Not really," he clucked. This was not the first time someone had asked him that question.

"Why not?"

"He has two problems," Bill began.

"Two?"

"Yes, two. He's too slow. He can't run with those guys in the NBA. He may even be too slow to play in Europe. And he's too white."

"Too white?"

"Sports jargon. White man's disease."

It was not a term she'd ever heard before.

It meant the inability to jump.

She knew what that meant.

"And he's too chicken. He is afraid to mix it up with the big boys."

"Just with little girls," she quipped.

"What?"

"Nothing." She thanked him and hung up.

So much for her favorite suspect.

On to her other suspects. The Krollers. They were Tom's territory. Tom! Another call. Another message.

She took the 'vette and drove to Glencoe to the Krollers' neighborhood. And drove around slowly.

A car was following her.

Should that frighten her? Or reassure her? Or both? Or neither? She was certain it wasn't Beth. So she didn't care who it was.

Very slowly.

Reading addresses. And names. Some mailboxes had names.

The Feldmans. The Joneses. Not worth keeping up with. The Collinses. Neighbors. Two blocks away. Mrs. Kroller had remembered them.

The Weavers.

They too still lived there. Leslie had remembered them.

She would make one more lap. On foot. And look in some of the mailboxes. And she did.

And found what she was looking for. The Russells. Mrs. Stephen Russell. Living right next door to the Krollers.

The eleventh witch.

A next-door neighbor.

For how long?

Long enough not to be remembered? Long enough to be suppressed. To be forgotten? To have been one of the witches?

There was one way to find out. Dennie looked over her shoulder. The car had stopped about a half block down.

Here goes. She walked up to the door and rang the bell.

A woman answered. She seemed to be in her sixties. Old enough.

"Mrs. Russell?"

"Yes."

"I just moved into the neighborhood. My name is Ward." It was the first name that popped into her head. It was a big improvement on Eller. She looked over her shoulder. The car was edging closer.

So was one of the Eller boys.

"Yes."

"How long have you lived here?" Why beat around the bush?

"Forty years."

Long enough.

The car stopped in front of the Russells. Mike got out and waved her badge at Eller. Everyone froze in place.

It was time to go home.

※※※※

When she drove by her apartment, there was a squad car parked out front. Tom's squad car. It had to be. But he was not inside the car. He had to be inside waiting for her.

She drove into the basement, parked the 'vette, and ran up the two flights of stairs.

He wasn't in the hall outside her apartment.

She opened the door.

He was inside.

"Darling," she said.

"Liar," he said.

Chapter
XV

"**D**arling," she repeated, closing the door behind her. How had he gotten inside her apartment?

"You lied to me!" he bellowed. There was no salutation. No greeting. No hug. No kiss. No warmth. Just an angry accusation that hung in the air long after Tom had emitted it.

"What do you mean?" Dennie demanded, becoming angry herself. Why was he treating her like this?

"I talked to Sean Keneally. He told me everything."

That was the reason. Dennie's anger dissipated more quickly than it had built up. Tom had a right to be mad at her. She had lied to him, And now Tom knew it. But did Tom really know everything? What had Sean told him? Everything? Did Sean know everything? Everything about Beth? And Jessie? Oh God.

"There are no three sisters. What a charade. This whole thing, from the cards to the name, to. . . . Sean told me. Not sisters. Sister. One sister."

Tom knew. Sean had told him her secret.

"You have only one sister. Not two. One. Why? Why did you have to lie to me?"

"Precisely what did Sean tell you?" she asked urgently.

"That you have only one sister. That Jessica doesn't exist. That Elizabeth doesn't exist. Neither of them. No. One of them does exist. Elizabeth, I suppose. Beth. And the other one isn't real. Jessie, she's . . . she's . . . whatever she is."

"They are both real," Dennie pleaded. How could he be so damn ignorant? Hold on. Don't be angry at him. It wasn't his fault. "Tom, you must believe that. You have to. Please. They both exist."

"Bullshit," he said eloquently.

"Tom, you don't mean that."

"Don't tell me what I mean."

"Don't be angry at her."

"Which one?"

"Beth."

"Is she the real one?"

"Be angry at me. I had to lie to you."

"You had to lie? Were you lying when we made love? Or only before and after?"

"I'm sorry I hurt you. I try hard not to hurt anyone I care for, but it's so damn difficult sometimes. I never want to hurt someone I love. But it seems that all I do is hurt people I love."

"So how many lovers have you hurt this way?" he demanded, needing to know.

"Lovers, or men I loved?" she asked him.

"Men you loved. Lovers. Is there a difference?"

"Yes. You know there is."

"What do you do, just hop into bed with guys right and left?"

"Damn it, Tom, stop it. I'm not just a girl you picked up in a bar."

"I'm sorry. I didn't mean all of that."

"Sure, I've had a few lovers. I never told most of them anything. They didn't matter. Not really."

"And men you loved?"

"One other."

"And you hurt him?"

"Yes, by never telling him anything. Until we no longer had anything left to share with each other."

"Tell me about her," Tom said with a deep sigh.

"Them," she reminded him. "Them."

"Them, then," he conceded.

"Sit down, please," she requested softly.

He did. In a chair in the far corner of the living room, as far away from the couch and her desk as possible. It was getting dark in the room. The sun was beginning to set. Dennie didn't turn on any lights. Or the TV. Or the CD. No illumination. No background noise. Just the two of them. And a truth that had to be addressed so that the two of them could continue to have something to share. She sat behind her desk.

They were now dissociated from one another. No longer lovers. Disconnected. Apart. She had to bring them back together. She couldn't let Beth and Jessie screw this one up. She couldn't screw this one up. She started with the simple idea that Beth and Jessie were both real. They both existed. He had to accept that much or they'd get no place at all.

That was asking a lot.

Please, for her sake. Try. Listen. Please.

He said that he would try.

"Please, try hard. Just don't judge until you've heard me out."

"Okay, I'll listen. But there was only one of them."

He had to accept that there were two. That Elizabeth and Jessica were two separate beings. They represented two different personalities. Two personalities existing in one body.

Whose body?

Beth's.

From the beginning?

No. Not from the very beginning. There hadn't always been two of them. At first she'd been no more than just an imaginary friend. Lots of kids had imaginary friends.

"Jessie had a friend?"

"No, Jessie was the friend." But then Jessie became more real. Less imaginary. More independent.

When?

Around age seven.

Why?

Dennie didn't know for sure.

What happened around then?

Dennie had no idea. It had happened to Beth. Not to her. And not all at once. Gradually.

"You have no idea?" he persisted.

"No."

"None at all?" doubtingly.

"No."

He let that subject drop.

As time passed, the two personalities both developed. They became more individual. Jessica became the formal one. Pristine. Proper. Aloof. Interested in science. And mathematics. And later, computers. Strong. Stern. Unapproachable.

And Beth. She was almost the opposite. She became a tomboy. She was interested in sports. And scouting. She was always dirty. Hated dresses. Never wore them. Jessie went to the school dances. Not Beth.

How?

Jessie pretended to be Beth.

This was getting too complicated for him.

And for poor Beth. The two personalities became totally separated. Complete dissociation into two separate personalities. That was, she informed him, the correct psychiatric terminology. Dissociation into multiple personalities. Two individual beings.

When?

By college.

"What did your parents think?"

"They were beside themselves. They were lost. They wanted her to get help. But they wouldn't. Beth and Jessie. Neither of them. Not as long as they were thought of as one person. Never. Then things got worse."

How could they have gotten worse?

"Mom died. Of cancer. In six weeks. Cancer of the pancreas. One day she was well. And then she was gone. And dad got sick. And then that guy tried to rape her."

"Beth?"

"No. He was on a date with Jessie. Or so he thought. And. . . ."

"And Beth was the one who stabbed him."

"Yes. Beth was tougher. Angrier."

"So that was why it was all hushed up. She really couldn't charge him with anything at all. Something might have come out."

"That's right. They were both frightened. So was dad. Fortunately, dad had enough connections."

"Sean Keneally."

"Among others."

"He wouldn't have needed many others."

"Dad made them enter therapy."

"Who went?"

"Beth. She entered therapy with Roger Nielsen. And Jessie. . . ."

"Had an affair with Sean."

"She acted out. She rebelled. Maybe she saw the handwriting on the wall. If Beth was getting treatment, it couldn't be good for her. She seduced Sean. It was her last desperate act. She was trying to save her own existence. Then dad died."

"After he set up Three Sisters Limited, so you could take care of both of them."

Tom was beginning to understand what she wanted him to understand. Needed him to understand. She needed his understanding and his love.

"And Beth got better. Thanks to Roger Nielsen." Her voice was less shrill now. More relaxed.

"So what happened to Jessie?"

"Poof. She disappeared. Beth no longer needed her. Beth was cured."

"But you still talk about Jessie as if she existed." He was still confused.

"She did. She and Sean were in love. Ask him."

"I did. That's what started all of this." Tom hesitated. "And you miss her?" He was still puzzled.

She nodded. It was the truth.

"Why this charade?"

"It isn't a charade. What was I supposed to do? Tell Beth that she was a psycho? A freak? That we were some modern version of 'The Three Weird Sisters' complete with eye of newt? I loved my sister. I still love her. Period. Every aspect of her. And I accept her. She misses part of her. And, damn it, so do I."

"And so does Sean. He told me as much."

"Tom, I need a hug."

He got up, crossed the room, stood in front of her. The room was very dark. He reached out with both hands, took her hands, and pulled her to her feet. They stood toe to toe only touching with their hands.

He dropped her hands and hugged her. In a full-blown bear hug.

"Tighter," she said.

His arms grasped her as tightly as he could.

She moaned softly and began to sway, rubbing herself against him, her breasts against his chest. Her lower abdomen against his loins. Slowly. Back and forth.

"I love you, Lieutenant Thomas Ward," she said.

"And I love you, Dennie, but I still have to talk to your sister."

"I know," continuing to move, but in a more rotary fashion.

"I'll be gentle with her."

More gyrations. He was not responding. Why not? Didn't her body turn him on? It had been good for him. Or it had seemed to be. Men didn't fake orgasms. Did they fake their intensity? The degree of their pleasure? All orgasms were not equal. Some were better than others. Some of hers sure were. And it was one of those better ones she wanted right now.

"You don't have to be that gentle." She slipped her hand in between them. He started to respond.

"All you women are the same. All you want to do is jump in the sack."

"I don't want to jump in the sack."

"You don't?"

"No. I want to make love. I want to make love to you. There's a big difference."

"You'd better go to the bathroom."

"I don't want to do it in the bathroom."

"Neither do I, but I don't believe in coitus interruptus."

She broke away from his hug. "Nor do I, not with you," and closed the bathroom door behind her.

She was in love.

✳✳✳✳

"Please don't ever lie to me again," Tom said.

"What choice did I have? She is my sister. I love her. I accept her. If she had cancer, would I desert her? I can't make her confront her problem. I have to show her my love. What else can I do?"

"It could destroy me."

They clung to each other furiously as his story tumbled out. It was a story made up of lies, deception, mendacity, centering on his wife. Correction. His ex-wife. And an affair with his best friend. Correction. His ex-best friend. Going on for a decade. Or more. The discovery. The taunting. The questions. Who was the father of *his* son? Impotence. Ridicule. Separation. Depression. Attempted suicide. Divorce. Psychotherapy. Work. Work. More work.

A woman. A new relationship. A new start. More like a rerun of a grade B movie. Lies. Impotence. Defeat.

And celibacy.

And more work.

Why hadn't he told her all of this?

It was his baggage.

"We both have baggage," she told him.

"Another lie could destroy me. Especially from you. I do love you, Dennie Cater."

"And I love you, Tom Ward."

"I can't go through that again," he told her. "I can't."

"You won't have to, no matter what. Because I love you, no matter what happens."

"What if I get depressed again?"

"I can deal with that."

"Impotent?"

"Yes, but I prefer it the other way."

"So do I."

"So let's prove you're not," she suggested.

✳✳✳✳

"So what happens next?" he asked.

"I catch my breath."

"To us."

"What do you want to happen?"

"I want to live happily ever after with you."

My God. He meant it. Happily ever after.

"So do I," she answered, surprising herself more than him. "But what about Beth? I have to help her. She's my sister. She's in such pain."

"Then we'll have to help her," he said.

"Are you sure you can do that?"

"For you. I can do that for you."

"No. Not for me. For us."

Chapter
XVI

A t precisely ten minutes to nine, Leslie arrived. Tom and Dennie were already there, waiting for her. One glance at her and Dennie knew she'd made the right decision. Leslie was almost beside herself. Her hair was not in place and her coat was buttoned wrong. She'd even neglected to put on any makeup. She was biting down hard on her lower lip and wringing out her gloves as if they were filled with water. This was not going to be easy on poor Leslie. Is it ever easy on the victim? Thank God Nielsen was as good as he was, even if he was opinionated. Or, as Slatter would have put it, biased. A Freudian to the end. Fantasy and wish fulfillment triumphant over any consideration of archetypal images. Nielsen might not believe in ritual satanic cults but he did believe in abused children. More important, he knew how to help such patients. Dennie introduced Tom and Leslie as if they were both old friends of hers who somehow had never met each other and then the three of them got into the elevator.

"He's cute," Leslie whispered anxiously in her ear. Dennie wasn't quite sure if that had been a question or an opinion. So she nodded. After all, he was, even though he was wearing the same clothes he'd worn yesterday. He had not expected to stay the night. She hoped he'd never make that mistake again. At least he'd showered. And shaved. With Beth's electric razor. The one she used on her legs. Share and share alike. Like good sisters.

Once the elevator deposited them on the eleventh floor, Tom rang the buzzer. It echoed down the hall and in less than a minute a nurse appeared and opened the door for them. Tom explained who they were. The nurse was expecting them. She put Leslie in Room 1108 and then showed Tom and Dennie into the room next to it, a room that had no number on its door, as if someone were trying to hide its existence as well as its purpose. As if that were somehow sinister. Like John Doran's hidden camera. The room itself was only dimly lit. Tom and Dennie sat down. Through the two-way mirror they could see Leslie waiting all by herself on the other side of the looking glass. Suddenly Dennie felt more like a voyeur than an interested friend, a professional observer. What were they doing to Leslie? Would this really help her? Or were they merely invading her privacy for their own purposes? Visitors to someone else's deflowering? Participants in a strange sort of emotional rape? Accessories? Like all those other witches? Dennie looked at Tom. If he had any such misgivings, he showed no evidence of them.

The door opened again. A woman came in. She was in her early thirties. Her appearance was striking. Why did some people think that word was an insult? Dennie didn't. The woman was tall and stood up straight, with a real presence. She had thin lips and light blue eyes. Both stood out in stark contrast to her jet black hair, which was cut so short that it emphasized the whiteness of her long pale neck and her long white coat. That was a symbol that Dennie understood.

"Hi," she said, introducing herself, "I'm Kris Swensen."

Dennie introduced herself and then Tom Ward. Kris Swensen shook hands with each of them. She had no pretensions. No insistence on "Doctor Swensen." Just a friendly manner and long elaborate earrings with a complex design of witches' hats, skulls, and broomsticks. Why had she picked out those earrings to wear? Although they did look good. With that neck and that hair and that posture, long, dark, dangling earrings were perfect. But why witches?

Kris Swensen saw Dennie staring at her earrings. "Wild, aren't they?" was all she said before telling them that a Mr. Keneally had called her. He said that he had to be in court. And asked her to relay the message.

The three of them sat down behind the mirror and waited. Dr. Nielsen should be there any moment now. He never kept patients waiting.

"This should be fun," Kris said. "Roger Nielsen and I talked about it yesterday morning. We went over the whole interview. Great stuff."

Fun was not the word Dennie would have used. Pain would have been closer, or torture. A ritual form of torture designed to get at the truth. Anything but fun. Look at Leslie. She was so damn nervous. She was still wringing out her gloves and biting her lips and looking around the room, avoiding the mirror. She looked so damn vulnerable.

"Roger is really excited. He went home early just so he could read up on witchcraft. I lent him several of my books. It's not a subject that most Freudian analysts have ever studied in any detail. He was really getting into it. He didn't know all the literature but I'm sure he does by now." She looked at her watch. "I wonder where he is?"

There was a knock on the door. It was Dr. Nielsen's secretary. He wouldn't be in until later.

"What are we going to do?" Dennie asked. "Poor Leslie, she's waiting to be interviewed by him. We can't just send her home. Look at her."

"I can interview her," Kris said, and before anyone could stop her she waltzed out of the room and appeared within the other room, the room on the other side of the looking glass. A voyeur transformed. Was that some form of obscene wish fulfillment? Or did she really know what the hell she was doing?

Leslie looked up at her and said something. What? They couldn't hear. Kris Swensen said something back to Leslie. The two of them shook hands with each other and Kris sat down. She was now very much the doctor. The presence in charge. She looked the part. Looks weren't everything. Dr. Swensen was now facing Leslie. She was seated on one side of the room; Leslie was sitting on the other side. And they were talking to each other. There had to be a switch somewhere.

Where?

On the wall, near the mirror. Dennie found it and flicked it.

"So, shall we get started?" Dr. Swensen asked. Her tone was friendly, informal.

"I guess so. Doctor . . . Doctor, I've forgotten your name already. I'm sorry."

"I know you're nervous. It's Swensen. Doctor Swensen. It's okay."

"Swensen," Leslie said to herself.

Kris smiled and nodded. Her earrings bounced. Leslie saw them and cringed.

Some fun. Even the earrings elicited terror. Terror bordering on panic. Like showing the victim the tools of torture before starting the questions. This is just the rack. Ignore it. No big deal. It's just for those who don't cooperate. Why the hell was she there? Why was Tom? Did he get into things like this? Questioning a suspect? Questioning a victim? Was there a difference? There had to be. Questioning Beth?

"Tell me about your dream, Leslie. Why don't we start there? I want you to remember your dream. If you can remember it, then you won't be afraid of it." Friendly and reassuringly.

"I know. We're only afraid of the unknown. That's what Mr. Doran told me. He was my therapist."

"And he was a good therapist." Even more reassurance.

"He was the best," Leslie told her, fighting back her tears. "No one else will be like him."

"Leslie, that's not true. He did help you. That's what good therapists do. But he was not unique. There are many other doctors who will be able to help you just as much."

Kris Swensen was good. Leslie was gaining confidence in her and as she did she began to relax. She had put down her gloves. And she was no longer biting her lip as she listened. Dennie could also hear a difference in Leslie's voice. And she could see it in her body.

Dennie reached across and squeezed Tom's thigh. He reached down and took her hand in his and squeezed it. She squeezed back. Thank God he was here with her.

"Tell me about your dream." More insistent this time, but still not demanding. A friend not a doctor.

Leslie started to answer. She hemmed; she hawed. She started; she stopped. And Kris Swensen kept bringing her back. Nudging her on. Prodding her ever so gently. And then slowly but surely the dream formed itself.

It was her dream about witches. Her dream of all dreams. The one that now had triumphed and recurred over and over again. That seemed to be gaining strength. Just when it should have been going away.

Where? Where were the witches?

In her backyard.

How could she be sure of that?

In the dream she saw her tree. Her own tree with her swing. The tree in her backyard.

This was familiar territory to Dennie but not, she realized, to Kris Swensen. Kris was starting from scratch. She knew all about witchcraft and satanic rituals, but she knew next to nothing about this patient. It was an initiation for both of them. Kris hadn't seen the tape.

Leslie described the tree and the swing vividly. Like a picture postcard from hell, Dennie thought.

Kris took a notebook out of the pocket of her long white coat and began to take notes. Notes of what Leslie was saying to her. A record of a trip to hell.

"Tell me about the witches," Kris said.

"What about the witches?" Hesitantly.

"How many were there?" A simple question.

"Twelve."

That was the same answer she had given Doran. An answer he hadn't accepted. Neither did Kris Swensen.

"Count again," Kris said.

"Twelve. Twelve and my mother."

"And how many did that make? How many altogether?"

"Thirteen."

The coven was collected. Now the ritual could begin.

"And what were they wearing? Those thirteen witches?"

"Gowns. Long gowns. Long black gowns."

"Was that all?"

"No."

"What else were the witches wearing?" Kris's questions remained gentle, asked like a friend, a helpful friend.

"Hats, black hats. Witches' hats. You know the ones. Shaped like ice cream cones only upside-down."

"What were they doing? Those thirteen witches in the long black gowns and the high black hats?"

"Dancing. They were dancing. All the witches were dancing."

"How?"

"Like witches danced. Dancing witches."

"And how is that?"

"In a circle. A witch's circle. A bunch of witches dancing in a big circle. They were all dancing in a big circle around me."

The ritual was in full swing.

"And what else? What else were they dancing around?"

"The tree. My tree. My own tree. The tree in my own backyard. The one I had a swing on."

It was almost as if it were the violation of that tree that hurt. It was her tree. In the same way that it was her body.

"Was that all they were dancing around?"

"No. No, there was something else."

"Something. What?"

She wasn't sure.

"Think back. Think harder. What could it be?"

She still wasn't sure.

"What did the witches dance around? Sometimes they danced around an altar. Could it be an altar?"

"What?"

"An altar. The witches could have been dancing around an altar."

"Yes, that was it."

Was she sure?

She was. It was an altar. The witches were dancing around an altar.

"What shape was it? This witches' altar."

Leslie wasn't sure.

"Smaller on top than on the bottom?"

"Yes. Yes. That was it. I can see it."

And Dennie could see her cringing.

"And the fire."

"Oh, God, the fire. How could I have forgotten that?"

"Tell me about that bonfire."

"The flames were so bright. And flickering. A big bonfire. The flames lit up their faces. The flames were orange. And yellow. Shining on their faces. They were dancing. We were dancing. We were all dancing around the bonfire. And the altar. And my tree."

"Was that the only fire?"

"The only fire? Yes."

Was she absolutely certain of that?

"No." She wasn't.

It was moving so quickly now. Leslie was remembering more and more details. More than she had even remembered for John Doran. There was no question about it. Dr. Swensen was good. She knew just what she was doing. It would help Leslie. Dennie was sure of that. She squeezed Tom's hand again. He again responded by squeezing back.

What else was burning? What else could be burning? Giving off light and heat, like a fire. Other fires? Candles?

Candles. Yes, there were candles.

A circle of candles?

Yes.

Black and white candles?

Yes.

But only one was white?

Only one white candle.

By now Dennie was squeezing Tom's hand for all she was worth. No wonder some therapists didn't believe these stories. All these trappings. Like a scene out of some bad Gothic novel. Or one of those old black and white B horror films. But these things did happen.

"Who is on the altar?" It was a question that had to be answered.

Leslie hesitated. And bit her lower lip. And twisted her hair in her hand.

"Who is she?"

"A woman."

"Is she dressed?"

"Dressed?"

"Or naked?"

"Naked. She's naked. The woman is naked."

"Is the woman just lying there? Naked? On the altar?"

"No."

Leslie was shivering now. She was shaking. So was Dennie.

"Tell me about her nakedness. Her exposed nakedness. Her helplessness. It will help you to describe it. I'm here to help you."

"She's exposed. Her legs have been spread apart."

"Widely apart?"

"As wide as possible. Tied open."

"What happened to her?"

"She was . . . was. . . ."

"Before that?"

"Before?"

"The blood."

"The blood," Leslie repeated. "The blood in the chalice. They poured it on her. They held her mouth open and made her drink it."

"She drank the blood from the chalice."

"Yes. She drank the blood from the chalice."

Leslie fell silent. She was exhausted. Beaten. Some fun.

"Leslie, we have to get to the climax of the ritual. The ritual must end. The woman must be violated."

"She was. Oh, God," Leslie was sobbing now. "She was." Crying, sobbing.

"How? How was she violated? What did they put inside of her? What? Think, what did they have?"

"I can't remember. I don't want to. Don't make me. Don't make me do it!"

"Do it."

"Don't make me! Please."

"Take the candle," firmly.

"The candle," obediently.

"The white candle."

"The white candle."

"Chant it."

"The white candle," she chanted.

A canticle of candles.

"Do it. Put it in her."

"Put it in her."

"And keep chanting." Once again as an order.

"The white candle," Leslie intoned.

"Put it in."

"The white candle," she chanted.

"Take it out."

"The white candle. Put it in. Take it out," Leslie chanted. Once. Twice. Three times.

"Now put the candle down."

Leslie made no response.

"Put the candle down." Kris paused for just a moment. "And tell me what is happening. Tell me what is happening to that naked woman. The one on the altar. Tied on the altar. Exposed to them all. Open waiting for them. For them to do whatever they want. She can't stop them. It's not her fault. Her legs are tied up. She can only wait there. For them to do what they want to do to her."

"They are raping her."

"Who?"

"The men."

"Are they ordinary men?"

"Ordinary men?"

"Or men with masks?"

"Men with masks," automatically.

"Goat masks."

"Goat masks," flatly.

Leslie slumped in her chair.

"Go on."

"I can't."

"You must," the doctor insisted. "Leslie, you must."

"No. No. Don't do it to me."

"What? Don't do what to you?"

"They are tying me down."

"What? Who is tying you down?"

"Tying me to the altar. Me. Them. The witches. My mother. She is holding me down. He is on top of me. He is pushing inside of me. She won't let go of me. My legs are being pulled apart. So far apart. So far apart. They are being pulled right off of me."

She was panting now. And sobbing. "He's inside of me."

"And what is he doing to you?"

What did she think he was doing?

"He is not making love to you."

"Not making love," Leslie repeated. More a chant than an answer.

"It is not his sex that is inside of you. Not his sex."

"Not his sex." All but a mantra.

"It is his hand."

"His hand," Leslie's voice echoed back.

"Pulling. Pulling."

"Pulling," automatically.

"Pulling something out."

"Pulling something out."

"Of you."

"Of me."

"From your womb."

"From my womb."

"Your baby."

"My baby."

"Your unborn baby."

"Aagh," Leslie screamed. It was a solitary piercing scream. A scream from the bottom of her soul. A scream like no other Dennie had ever heard. A scream that filled the room. Both rooms. A scream of terror. Of pain. Of suffering. The mother of all screams. A scream that could be both felt and heard.

"Aagh," again.

And then Leslie slumped in her chair and passed out.

"Aagh," the scream continued. The scream of terror. Of pain. "Aagh."

Leslie had fainted but her scream had not ended. It had a life of its own. It was no longer her scream. Not Leslie's.

It was Dennie's own voice. She was screaming. "Aagh!" Tom touched her shoulder. "It happened. It all really happened," Dennie shouted.

He put his arms around her.

She screamed again. "The fucking son of a bitch. He did it to her."

Tom hugged her.

"He did that to his own little girl."

Chapter
XVII

Dennie continued to scream. Tom's hugging was not helping to calm her down. Her voice had a life of its own. A meaning. A source. A half scream made up of all of her terrors. God, there had been so many. She'd been mugged. Then someone had tried to kill her. His strength was there for her. To lean on. To rely on. He was there for her. Her screaming stopped. She was now panting hard. Fighting for her breath. Finding it. She could feel her entire soul trembling. Could he? He had to. He kissed her once on the forehead. Not out of lust. Anything but lust. He could never treat a woman like that. Or a suspect. Not her. Not Beth. She had almost caught her breath. Her heart was merely pounding now.

The light went on inside the room and when it did Dennie could no longer see through the mirror. Leslie had disappeared from her view. Poor unconscious Leslie. Dennie hoped that she was feeling no pain now. Was she still inside the world behind that looking glass? Or would she wake up in terror? No, she wouldn't. She hadn't before. Leslie had been through her dream before. With Doran. Not quite like this, but pretty darn close. And then she'd gotten up and gone to school. Or home. Or whatever. How could people do that? She had no idea. But they did. Taking their own looking glasses with them. And their private terrors.

The door opened, and Kris Swensen strode into the room. "That was hard work," she said. "A lot harder than I thought it would be. And a heck of a lot more fun, too."

"Fun!" Dennie was incensed. "How can you say that that was fun! It was anything but fun!"

"Take it easy," Kris said.

"Take it easy! Poor Leslie. That poor kid!"

"Yes. Poor Leslie. I wish Roger Nielsen were here. She needs his help. She has been abused alright. No doubt about that. Terribly abused. But not in the way you think. She was abused by her therapist. That guy ought to have his license yanked. If he has one."

"Abused by her therapist? By John Doran?" Dennie couldn't believe that. Doran had helped her. "What the heck are you talking about?"

189

"She's a very vulnerable girl. More like a little girl than a young woman. It's hard to believe that she's almost twenty. She is both vulnerable and suggestible. Very suggestible."

"Suggestible!"

Why wasn't Tom saying anything? He'd heard what she had heard. Seen what she'd seen. Was he so damn callous? Maybe he did treat witnesses like that. An emotional third degree. "Tom?"

He shrugged, noncommittally.

"Here," Kris Swensen said, taking a sheet of paper out of her notebook. "Here, take this. These are my notes. My notes of everything you just witnessed, in the order that it took place."

Kris tried to hand the piece of paper to Dennie. Dennie didn't reach out for it.

"I don't need your notes. I heard what Leslie went through."

"Take them," Dr. Swensen ordered her.

"I won't."

"Dennie, please," Tom requested.

Was he on her side? Or on Dr. Swensen's? Didn't he care about Leslie? About her?

"Do what the doctor is asking you to do. I think it must be important," he explained.

"It is," the doctor reiterated, still holding out the slip of paper toward her.

The doctor! Trying to look so damn important. With those stupid earrings dangling halfway to the floor. Some shrink. As sensitive as a Brillo pad. Dennie took the damn sheet of paper. What choice did she have? They were ganging up on her. She looked out toward the other room but still could not make out Leslie. Poor little Leslie. Had she just gotten up and gone home? What the hell. She'd been raped by her stepfather. And now by some stupid shrink. Small potatoes. Things like that happened everyday. Just close your legs, get off your back, pull your clothes back on, and go about your business. You can't get AIDS from this kind of rape. Small consolation, that.

"Read it," Kris Swensen said. "Out loud. One item at a time. And remember what you saw and heard. Exactly what you witnessed. And think about each item. Did I record them correctly? Is that what Leslie really remembered? What she described to me? And are my notes in the right order? Do they really reflect the session? Is that what really happened in that little room?"

"I know what happened. Do you?" Dennie countered.

"Dennie, please," Tom's voice sounded concerned. Maybe he cared.

"Think about the order," Dr. Swensen said again. So damn officiously.

"The order! What difference does that make. Who cares which came first? The rape or the blood? Who cares?"

"I care. And you will, too. It is all that matters. It is pivotal. It's what really happened."

"Pivotal! All that matters! Get real. What matters is what happened to your patient."

"Read."

Dennie read. "The first line says 'witches.' 'Witches.' That's all. Just one word." This was going to get them absolutely no place. It was worse than reading a play-by-play of a game that had ended. And that your team had lost.

"Well," the doctor asked.

Damn it, she wasn't the patient here.

"Dennie." Said so damn sweetly. As if he did care.

"That seems right. The first thing was the witches. No, wait, she started with her tree. Her tree and her swing."

"Yes, she did, but the first satanic part, the first part of the satanic ritual that Leslie mentioned, was the witches."

Dr. Swensen was right. Dennie would give her that one. The dream had started with the witches. "That's right."

"Read on."

"Thirteen," Dennie said.

"The number of witches," Tom agreed. "Twelve plus her mother. A coven."

"Thirteen," Dr. Swensen said.

"Black," Dennie read. "Black gowns. Long black gowns."

"Their clothing," Tom said. "That's what they wore."

"And then the hats," Dennie went on. "The high black hats that looked like upside-down ice cream cones."

"Continue."

She did.

"The dancing. The witches all dancing in a circle. Around the altar. Then came the fire." Dennie was now linking together the words of the list, adding descriptive phrases. But she realized she was not changing the order. She added details to the narrative, but those details did not change the order in which things had happened.

Kris stopped her. "Is that what you both heard? In just that order?"

They both thought so.

She had Dennie read from the list again. Word for word.

"Witches. Thirteen. Black gowns. Witches' hats. Dancing. Circle. Altar. Fire."

The three of them agreed. That was the order of the dream. The ritual. The order of Leslie's satanic ritual.

Of course the order mattered. This was a ritual. It had to follow a specific order. All rituals did. It was the order that proved its authenticity. It was proof positive. Dennie went back to the scribbled notes. There had been candles. Black candles and white candles. But only one white candle. And there was a woman on the altar.

Naked.

Legs splayed apart.

Violated.

No, not yet.

She'd been forced to drink blood from a chalice. Then she'd been violated.

"How?" Kris asked.

Candles.

Men.

Men in goat masks.

Was that the proper order?

Yes. Tom was certain of that. So was Dennie. There were some things you never forgot.

Had she left anything out so far?

No.

Had she added anything?

No. Neither of them thought that she had added anything.

"Finish the list," she said.

Dennie read the last two entries. "Abortion. Fetus." The words somehow did not actually express what she had heard.

"Well?" Kris asked.

"Okay," Dennie admitted. Although abortion sounded so sterile. So medical. Ripped from her own womb. Like MacDuff. Only too early to live. Ripped out to be killed. Sacrificed. Eaten.

"Tom?"

He had nothing to add.

"Do you both agree that this is the ritual that Leslie described to me? In the exact order that she described it? This is her ritual. The ritual of her dream. The story she told me. The story you heard her tell me." With that Kris took the list and read it aloud once again.

"Witches. Thirteen. Black gowns. Witches' hats. Dancing. Circle. Altar. Fire. Candles. Black and white. One white candle. A woman. Naked. Legs apart. Violated. Not yet. Blood. Chalice. Violation. Candles. Men. Men in goat masks. Abortion. Fetus."

"Are we all in agreement?"

"Yes," Dennie insisted. "Of course we are."

"Look on that desk behind you."

Dennie did. There was a single typed sheet of paper on it.

"I put that there before I left the room to interview her. Read it."

Dennie grabbed the sheet of white paper. All it contained was a list of words. She started to read it. "Witches. Thirteen. Black gowns. Witches' hats. Dancing. Circle. Altar. Fire. Candles. Black and white. One white candle. A woman. Naked. Legs apart. Violated. Not yet. Blood." She stopped. What was this?

"Finish it."

"Chalice. Violation. Candles. Men. Men in goat masks. Abortion. Fetus. I don't understand."

"No. You understand. You just don't want to accept what you understand. Dr. Nielsen and I put that list together yesterday. It's pretty much what you and I had discussed on the phone. The entire satanic ritual rigamarole. That was the story Dr. Nielsen was going to get her to tell to him. To us. He couldn't get here so I took over and got the same story. She didn't tell you that fable. I did. That dream did not come from Leslie. It came straight out of the mind of her therapist."

"John Doran."

"That charlatan," Kris said.

"But all these kids have been molested. And sacrificed. And killed. It wasn't all lies. It couldn't be. Could it? Tom, help me. You're a cop. You're a homicide cop. You must know all about these kinds of ritual murders."

"There are no ritual murders. None," the doctor contradicted her.

"None?"

"That's always been the hooker. There's never been any physical evidence. We hear all of these stories. Hundreds of them. Thousands even. Who knows how many? And yet there is never any proof at all. Not even a shred of physical evidence. No blood. No bodies. Nothing."

"Nothing? How could that be?" Dennie asked.

"It couldn't be. That's the point. You'd have to believe that there are some very powerful creeps who are going around the country and killing people as part of some satanic ritual and getting away with it. Time after time after time. It's possible, I guess. But I don't believe it. The number of cases has been growing and growing. We now have hundreds of victims. All telling the same story. Different places. Different years. Different parts of the country. From Maine to Montana. But the stories are always the same. If you put them together, then thousands of warlords, or warlocks, or satans, or whatever have murdered untold thousands of people, and gotten away with it. Year after year after year. Clean. Scot-free. And there is just no damn evidence. None, and I mean that literally. No bodies. And, what's more, no witnesses. No participants. Not one. Not one person has ever left a satanic cult and then blown the whistle on them.

"Nobody has ever turned in a single warlock. People even testify against the mafia. Hell, the devil himself couldn't have more power in this country."

"No one at all?" plaintively.

"Not one person."

"But with all these victims it must be true."

"Just the opposite," Tom told her.

"But there are so many victims, and they all tell the same story. I . . . I. . . ." Dennie didn't want to believe them.

"Dennie, you can't ignore the lack of physical evidence," Tom insisted.

"Lack. . . ."

"The doctor is right," Tom continued. "No bodies. No blood. Nothing. Not a single bloody chalice. Or blood-stained candle. And nobody has ever turned state's evidence. Wanted out and told a credible story. Nobody."

"But how could they all tell the same story?" Dennie pleaded.

Tom turned to Kris Swensen to answer this one.

"Lots of people tell the same story about being abducted by aliens. Bright lights. Flying saucers. Being taken up into spacecraft. A cop can't take a piss in the street today without some good citizen catching it on video. But there's not one video of an alien. Or of a UFO. It's almost as if they're allergic to video cameras. If we had enough camcorders, there were be no more aliens. The true Star Wars defense."

"Were they all lying?"

"Was Leslie?" Kris asked. "Was she lying?"

Poor Leslie. "No."

Dennie turned again to Tom. "Are you positive about that? That there are no ritual sacrifices?"

"I am," Tom assured her.

"And no ritual murders?"

There was a knock on the door. It was Roger Nielsen's secretary, obviously distraught.

"What's wrong?" Kris asked her.

"It's Dr. Nielsen. Poor Dr. Nielsen. He was murdered."

"Murdered!" Tom said.

"Yes. When he didn't get here, I got worried. I called his home. There was no answer so I. . . ."

At that moment Mike O'Rourke arrived. "Tom," she said, "you're needed."

"What's up?"

"I got a preliminary report from the cop on the beat. He said that Nielsen was stabbed. With a butcher knife."

"Oh, my God," Dennie gasped.

"And that's not all. His body was surrounded by a circle of black candles. And in his mouth there was one candle. A white candle."

"But that's impossible," Dennie said.

"Why?"

"Because there are no satanic ritual murders. Such things never happen. Didn't you know that?"

Chapter
XVIII

As they were pulling up to her apartment, Tom asked Dennie if it were alright with her if he came back in a couple of hours. That meant around two. Two in the afternoon was as good a time as any other, she told him. It really wasn't, but a girl could not always pick the time. It was picking the partner that counted, and she'd already done that. "I know why you want to come to my place," Dennie remarked, hope springing eternal.

"No, I don't think you do."

"I was afraid of that."

"I want to see all four of the tapes."

"I knew we'd be up all night."

"Cut it out, Dennie. Our love isn't everything."

Love, their love. Not their passion. Not their lust. Not their making love. Their love. He'd said that. Not the physical act, but the emotional state. Not the ritual, but its meaning. Its basis.

"Before I come by get some rest. It may be a long night," he said without a hint of a double meaning. "I'm going to have the tap taken off your phone, and the trace."

"Why?"

"I have to see Beth. I have to interview her. I'm going to tell Sean Keneally that the tap and trace are off your phones. That way he can tell her to call you or Mike. And when she calls you, we can arrange for a meeting. You can even be there if that's what Beth wants."

"I don't know if Beth will even call. Either me or Mike. I'm so worried about her. So is Mike. She thought Beth was saying goodbye to her. Not just goodnight, but more like a last farewell. A last goodnight. I don't know what she's thinking. Maybe she's leaving town or . . . something. Beth may be in some sort of trouble."

"She wouldn't leave town without saying goodbye to you, would she?" he asked.

"I don't know. Not under normal circumstances. But these have not been exactly normal circumstances. I have no idea what is going on in her head."

"I don't think she'd do anything desperate without talking to you," he said, trying to be reassuring.

"Maybe you're right. I don't know, I'm just so worried about her. She thinks she can take care of herself. But she can't. Not always. This may be way over her head." Her lower lip was quivering. She rolled it inward to hide the quivering.

"I'll pick you up outside your place at two," he said.

"Pick me up?" Dennie was confused. She thought he was coming over.

"We'll have a couple of chores to do before we watch those tapes."

"You knew there were four all the time, didn't you?" she asked him.

"Yes," he replied. He'd seen the four of them in Doran's office waiting to be taken. He couldn't take them because of the restraining order.

"Then why did you say there was only one. Were you testing me?"

"Maybe. Maybe I just didn't think they were very important."

"And I failed your test."

"I wouldn't say that."

Dennie got out of the unmarked squad car. "I love you, Tom Ward," she said.

"Two sharp," he said, looking straight ahead out of the windshield. The sun was bright. It was in the low forties. She'd have to remember her sunglasses. The sky was clear, light blue. A great day, a harbinger of a change of season? In Chicago you never knew until they'd already changed. "So you set me up."

"I did what?"

"You left the tapes there."

"Because I had to."

"And set me up."

"Let's say we're even."

"Don't ever do that again."

Tom still suspected Beth. That thought jarred Dennie. Setting her up was bad enough. Testing her. But thinking that Beth was a murderer. A cold-blooded murderess. Her own flesh and blood. Her lip was now quivering from anger. "Beth didn't kill anybody," she shouted at him.

"You don't know that and I don't know that."

"I know she didn't. I know her."

"And I know that there aren't any satanic ritual murders, but it's hard to prove that to Roger Nielsen."

✸✸✸✸

Tom was precisely on time. She liked a man who was prompt, and a woman, even a sister. Promptness was one of the few words that was not in Beth's vocabulary. That was one of the aspects that had made Jessie so nice. Jessie had always been on time. Although Beth had been better the last couple of years. As she had reincorporated Jessie. Some of Jessie's characteristics had broken through. Some of the nicer ones. Like promptness. And neatness. And orderliness. Not too much of that, but some.

Reincorporated. Was that the correct psychiatric term for it? It was dissociation that was the term. Un-dissociation. De-dissociation. Associate. Reincorporate. Poor Beth.

Tom drove up in the same car. He did not get out or make any move at all. Who said chivalry wasn't dead? Dennie opened the door all by herself and stepped into the front seat, beside him. He didn't even say hello but just put the car into gear and pulled away from the curb. It didn't handle quite like her 'vette.

"Where we going, my love?" she asked.

"What'd you do?"

"I called Beth and gave her your message. Isn't that what you wanted me to do?"

"I knew you knew where she was all the time."

"Stop this car," she ordered. "Right here."

He did. Right in the middle of the street. Dennie got out, slamming the car door behind her and started walking back to the entrance of her building, glancing back at him after taking half a dozen angry strides.

He had not moved a muscle. He was sitting there in the damn car doing nothing, like a lump of clay. As unresponsive to her needs as he'd been when they had started to make love that first time. But this was far worse. Who cared about the other? Sometimes it was good; sometimes it wasn't. And good was better than not so good. But it was all pretty much irrelevant. It took care of itself. But, damn it, she needed him emotionally.

She was really pissed off. For some unfathomable reason she thought he'd be different. A car honked as it pulled around Tom's car and suddenly he leaped into action. Like that moment he'd slipped his finger inside of her and had felt the diaphragm and come to life. One simple piece of latex in front of her womb. . . .

Ripped untimely from a mother's womb. The analogy shook her. Goddamn men. The hell with all of them. Beth had made the right choice. Not for the different way of making love but the different meaning of love itself. Mike never treated Beth like this.

Tom threw the car into reverse and the tires squealed as he drove back to intercept her. When he got between her and the entrance to her apartment, he slammed on the brakes and jumped out of the car.

Macho crap! Why couldn't he just apologize and tell her how much he loved her and that he doesn't know how to handle it and that he's scared. That he doesn't want to screw up this one.

He was standing in front of her now. She looked straight at him and could read nothing. A cold, indifferent nothing. Here it comes.

"Denise Cater," he began. "I love you. More than I ever loved anyone else. I'm sorry. It's . . . just . . . well. I apologize. I just don't know how to manage it. I'm so damn afraid I'll screw this up and lose you. I can't lose you. It's so damn complicated. I. . . . "

Her emotions melted away. Her anger. Her fear.

"Please forgive me," he pleaded.

"I was only making a bad joke. About calling Beth. Can't you tell? I'm scared, too." More frightened than he could possibly know.

"I know. You're frightened for Beth."

"Not just that. I'm also frightened for me. For us. I've never thought in terms of an 'us' before. I don't want to lose that. But what happens to us if Beth. . . ?" By now she was fighting back her tears.

"She couldn't have," Tom said.

"Why not?"

"She's your sister."

They both understood that as nice as that sounded and felt, it was not an adequate explanation for either of them. A killer could easily be someone's sister. Bonnie had been someone's sister. So had Lucrezia Borgia. And Ma Barker.

✳✳✳✳

As Tom drove northward along Lake Shore Drive, she told him what she'd done in the last two hours. Not because he'd asked her again. He hadn't. Or because he was a cop investigating a murder. Just because she wanted to share everything with him. The best reason of all.

First she had called Leslie English and given her the three names that she'd gotten from Dr. Slatter. What followed had been a series of questions, all of which reflected Leslie's anxiety and desperation. Who was Slatter? Did Dennie know anything about the three therapists? She didn't. Which one was better? Could Slatter be trusted?

Dennie tried her best. At least Slatter thought that John Doran was an excellent therapist. She didn't mention his comment as to Doran's unavailability. That Leslie already knew.

But which of them was the best?

She'd just have to pick one.

She would. And half an hour later, Leslie called her back. She had called one and would be seeing her that afternoon. Around five.

Dennie had told her that she hoped that would work out. She said the same thing to Tom. She hoped the new therapist could take up where Doran left off and help Leslie. Dennie also wondered whether this new therapist would be willing to testify for Leslie.

Was that important to Dennie?

No. Not really. She no longer cared. The major issue was helping Leslie and surviving. Leslie's therapists didn't have long life expectancies.

Which brought them back to John Doran and Roger Nielsen.

According to Tom, they had both been killed with the exact same type of butcher knife. From Ace Hardware.

"The place," she said, chanting a TV ad.

"Yes."

"So anyone could have bought them."

"Even Pat Summerall," Tom said.

"Who?"

"Or John Madden."

"Are they suspects?"

"You are precious."

"i hope you think so."

"They do the ads for Ace. Summerall played in the NFL. He was a defensive end and a place kicker. For the old Chicago Cardinals before they moved to St. Louis, and then for the New York Giants. Madden was coach in the NFL. For Oakland before they moved to L.A."

His explanation meant nothing to her. "So they aren't suspects."

"They're announcers," a bit exasperated.

"I see. And all announcers are innocent."

"Professional bystanders."

She assumed that meant that they weren't suspects.

They were at Belmont Avenue. Tom pulled off Lake Shore Drive and headed away from the lake and onto Belmont. She hadn't even enjoyed the view. And she always liked looking at the lake and the beaches. And the skyline. Especially on a bright, clear day. She'd been looking at Tom and enjoying the view.

Tom was talking. Saying very important things. Those lips did such important things. They couldn't trace the knife.

Or the candles.

And there were no fingerprints. There often weren't on a wooden knife handle. But the candles were also clean. Wiped clean.

All very professional, she suggested.

Perhaps.

No physical evidence, she concluded.

Right, he agreed.

Just like all of the other cases of ritual satanic abuse.

Except for one thing, he reminded her.

What was that?

This time there was a body.

A subtle difference, she grudgingly admitted. A mere detail. She told him that she had left messages for Beth. With Sean. On Mike's machine. On the answering machine of Three Sisters Limited.

She'd gone out and called in.

She could have changed the message.

What?

The recorded message. She could have changed that.

She hadn't thought of that.

He had. And he had asked Mike to change hers. And she had said she would. Did that mean there would be no more Harry Carey?

It did.

Good did sometimes come out of evil.

✳✳✳✳

Tom parked the squad car in an illegal spot. There were some advantages to being a cop. He got out and went around the car and opened the door for her. Chivalry was still breathing.

"What are we doing?" she asked.

"We're talking to Robin Riegel and then to your friend Brian."

"He's no friend of mine."

"He's lucky he hadn't gotten it out of his pants."

"Why?"

"Mike might have shot it off."

Like Beth had wanted to cut it off that guy who had tried to rape her, she thought. She was glad she hadn't said that.

Tom had called Robin and told her to wait for them in her apartment. They walked up to the third floor. The door had double locks. They were old and painted over and intact. Brian had not broken in. That much was obvious.

What else was obvious?

Tom rang the buzzer.

Robin was home. She had been expecting them. She asked them in. They sat in the small all-purpose front room, cluttered with old furniture, books, and knickknacks. Tom wasted no time getting down to details. This was not a social visit. How had Brian Havergal gotten into her apartment?

He'd been invited in. By Robin herself.

To her apartment only?

Yes, only into the sitting room.

Not into her bedroom?

Well, maybe. They'd gone in there to watch TV.

What was on TV that they wanted to watch in her bedroom?

Something.

Who wanted to watch it?

She did. Then he did it. He raped her. Tore her dress. She still had it. She could show it to them. She did. It was torn.

What time was that?

About eleven.

Tom nodded. Then what happened?

He did it again.

When?

About two.

When did he leave?

She didn't know. She'd gone to sleep.

Was she going to press charges?

No. The publicity would be terrible. Her parents were so . . . so . . . . From a small town. Catholic. It would kill her mom. She couldn't. Thank God she wasn't pregnant. She was on the pill.

✳✳✳✳

Brian told them pretty much the same story that Robin had. Only differently. Robin had started it all. She'd initiated everything. He hadn't started the ball rolling. She had. She had invited him into her bedroom. And once they got there, she, well, if they had to know, went down on him.

What about the torn dress?

It got torn in the excitement. Things like that happen.

"Mr. Havergal," Tom said, "you have your story. She has hers. All in all, we probably can't charge you."

"You can't prove nothing."

"But we can do one thing."

"What's that?"

"If I ever hear another story like Robin's, I'm going to hold it out and let Mike shoot it off."

"Fuck you!"

Tom punched him viciously right in the groin. Once.

Big Brian collapsed in agony with a scream. "Aaagh . . . I . . . You. . . ." He continued to scream and pant, doubled over in pain. "I'm . . . going to . . . file . . . a complaint."

"This witness saw nothing."

"She's a cop!"

"I'm the woman you jumped yesterday."

"Shit."

"After Mike shoots it off, I'll kill you," she added.

They left. "Where we going now?" she asked.

"Glencoe," Tom replied.

"The Krollers?"

"Their neighbors."

"The Russells?"

"The Russell. Mrs. Ewell Russell. He's dead."

"The forgotten witch," she said.

Chapter XIX

Mrs. Russell was also expecting them, but unlike either Robin Riegel or Brian Havergal, she had done something to prepare for their visit. She'd made fresh coffee and baked some pecan rolls. It was so tragic, what had happened to poor Billie. She was glad to help their investigation in any way she could but she had no idea how she could. Poor little Billie.

While Mrs. Russell was pouring the coffee, Dennie excused herself and went to the bathroom and took advantage of the phone in the hallway and called her answering machine. Beth had not called in. Or if she had, she had not left a message.

By the time Dennie got back to the living room, the coffee was poured and Mrs. Russell was passing out her homemade, fresh, hot pecan rolls. Dennie realized she hadn't eaten all day. She took two. They weren't that big. The living room was not as big as the Krollers' but whose was? And not as cold and austere. It wasn't the difference in size. Or decor. This was a room real people had lived in. Spilled coffee in. And tears. Real life.

Tom explained that they were interested in Billie Kroller's past.

She had heard that his death had. . . . Well . . . that he had . . . killed himself.

That was true.

She would tell them anything that they wanted to know.

What could she tell them about Billie Kroller?

He'd been a pretty normal kid, all things considered.

What all things?

His father.

Did she think that William Kroller was a problem?

"Yes," she said firmly.

Dennie was all ears. William Kroller was her prime suspect. The murder of Roger Nielsen could have been arranged by him. There was no evidence to follow up. Nothing that could be traced. Ordinary candles. A common butcher knife. To her that seemed more professional than coincidental. Just the witchcraft trappings. And that could all be nothing more than a set of red herrings.

"What about his father?" Tom asked, taking full charge of the questioning.

He was always mean to Billie. Mean and cold and distant. As if he didn't like him.

And to Leslie?

He worshiped her. He loved that little girl. Adored her. That was why this lawsuit was so tough on him.

Not exactly the image of a child molester. But what was? Did the neighbors really know? Hell, often the wife didn't. Or didn't want to. But Mrs. Kroller may have helped him.

And Mrs. Kroller?

Who could tell with her? She never showed her feelings. Her emotions. She must have had some. Everyone did. Did anyone want more coffee?

They both did.

Another pecan roll?

Tom did. He took one. Dennie wanted to do the same. She didn't. Two was enough. On second thought. No second thoughts allowed.

Mrs. Russell knew the whole story.

What whole story?

About the witchcraft, she told them. And the Black Sabbaths. Everything. She smiled and took a bite of her pecan roll. "They are good," she admitted.

Who was behind it?

Her husband. The late Ewell Russell. His friends had all called him Reb. That was short for Rebel. They were both from Richmond.

When had he died?

Two years ago.

They were so sorry.

She didn't seem to be.

"He organized the coven?" Dennie asked, taking the lead.

"What coven?" Mrs. Russell asked her.

"The coven of witches. A coven is a gathering of thirteen witches."

"I know what a coven is, but there was no coven of witches here in Glencoe. Not that I ever heard about. What an idea. Do such things really exist?"

"But I thought you said that your husband was behind it all."

"I did. But I wasn't talking about any real coven of witches. Nothing that outlandish. We had parties. In our backyard. Around a big bonfire. Annual costume parties. Every Halloween. Everyone came as witches. That was the rule. His rule. No pirates with eye patches. No presidential masks. Maybe a few ghosts. No Frankensteins. Dracula was always an open question. Just about everyone came as witches. Witches and their consorts. Warlocks. Not that anyone knew how a warlock looked."

Did all the neighbors come to those parties?

A lot of them did. Different ones came to different parties.

The Felsches? Had they come to the parties?

Yes.

Often?

Every year. They were regulars. He loved it. So did Mrs. Felsch.

The Williamses?

Yes, before the accident. That was such a tragedy.

Dennie said nothing.

And Collinses? Bergers? Risbergs?

Three more affirmative replies. The coven was gathering. Right there in Glencoe. At an annual Halloween party. This was not exactly the Black Sabbath that she'd expected to hear about.

And, of course, the Krollers?

Yes.

With Leslie?

Of course. And Billie. A lot of the kids came. They loved it. A costume party with adults. And a big bonfire. Lots of excitement.

Were there ever any rituals?

Mrs. Russell wasn't sure what she meant by rituals.

Dennie spelled it out for her. "Satanic rituals."

Those were performed by Stephen's friends, she said. With more than a trace of disdain in her voice.

What kind of rituals?

The usual type of satanic rituals. They even had all the symbols.

Such as?

They drank fake blood. It was some sort of red Kool-Aid, she thought.

From chalices?

Most certainly from chalices. And flagons. That was what made it into blood. The kids all loved that. Drinking blood from the great big chalices and dancing around the great big bonfire. Good clean fun.

Was there an altar?

Yes.

Did it ever get out of hand?

What did she mean?

With the kids?

No. Never. No one ever touched the kids. Not in her house.

With women?

Women?

Naked women? That's what usually happened on the altars. Women were stripped and . . . violated.

She laughed.

What was so funny?

Her husband's friends never touched a naked woman. Not with a ten-foot pole. Or anything else. Not in that way. They were all fags.

Fags.

So was he. He'd died of AIDS. And she was HIV positive.

Neither of them had any idea what to say to her.

She went on without waiting for them to say anything. She could guarantee that no women had been violated while people danced around that bonfire. Never. That was a sure bet.

No violation of anyone?

None whatsoever.

Except her. And her whole life. But not in the way they meant.

✳✳✳✳

Neither one of them said very much as they started to drive back to the city.

"Where are we going?" she finally asked.

"Your place," he said. "I want to watch some TV."

"That's what they always say."

He said nothing in reply.

"Robin asked Brian to watch TV with her and then look what she did to him. You can't trust women."

"All I want to do is watch those tapes."

Her attempt at humor had failed. She'd never been good at that type of banter. She didn't know what else to say. And she didn't like his emphasis on the *all*.

✳✳✳✳

There was a message waiting for her.

"Hi," the voice began.

"Beth," she said.

"Beth," he echoed.

"Shush," she elaborated.

"I'll be at that Mexican joint on Halsted just off Maxwell at one A.M. Tell that cop he can meet me there. But please don't come with him. Please. For my sake."

Click.

Beep. Beep. Beep.

"What a dump," he said. "Even the derelicts avoid that joint. How does she even know it exists?" Then he answered his own question. "Lots of cops go there. Mike probably took her there once."

Dennie had no idea. "Will you go alone?"

"Yes. But don't you want. . . ."

"I can't go. She doesn't want me there."

"Why?"

"I don't know."

Tom checked in. Mike was there. She had heard from Beth. She'd left a message. She would meet Tom alone at one at that. . . .

Tom had already gotten that message.

"Alone, Tom," Mike reminded her superior.

"I know."

"She means it."

"Was anything else new?"

The autopsy on Nielsen had been completed. He'd died of a single knife wound. That was not news. Between four and five the previous afternoon. That was.

Who the hell had been in his home at four in the afternoon?

Much of what had happened was now pretty clear. Whoever it was had not broken in. There was no evidence of forced entry. The best bet was that Roger Nielsen had let his murderer in.

Who? And why?

Those were questions Mike could not answer.

What about the fax?

It had been sent from Nielsen's own machine. When? At around four thirty. But the secretary got it at nine the next morning.

No, she got in at nine. There was a difference. The fax was already there. Waiting for her.

Did the murderer send it? And if so, why?

Mike had no idea. Nor did Tom. Nor did Dennie.

They had six hours until. . . . "Just enough time," he said.

That's just what she thought.

To watch the tapes. The four tapes from Doran's office.

He had known all along that there had been four. That meant that she had been set up by him. Neither of them said anything.

They started with the videotape of the late John Johnston, also known as the late Billie Kroller. Which of them had committed suicide? What a strange question. It was a convincing performance. Worthy of Anthony Perkins. Or Montgomery Clift. It sure as hell convinced the two of them that Billie had not known about the camera until that very day. That very moment.

Could he have killed Doran? they asked each other. In a rage. A premeditated rage. Precipitated by his discovery of the betrayal.

Yes, they both answered.

Did he have the opportunity? Yes. He could have gotten out of the locked unit. He got out the next day. To save her life. What about motive? Doran had betrayed him. Not with notes, but with videotapes. Lies. Sex. Videotapes. And betrayal. A deadly combination.

It was the videotapes that counted. Videotapes his dad might uncover. By mistake. By accident. Serendipity. While trying to get Leslie's. While going through Doran's files trying to uncover Leslie's and instead coming up with Billie's.

Did Billie know that Leslie was also Doran's patient?

He might have seen her there. Or talked to her about him. Had he? Ever? There was one easy way to find out. Dennie called Leslie. Did she know her half brother had been a client of Mr. Doran?

No, but she wasn't surprised. She'd recommended Doran to him the last time they' talked.

When was that?

Six months ago, she guessed.

That meant that Billie knew that John Doran was Leslie's therapist. So once he figured out the taping bit, he realized that there was a risk his dad might get hold of those tapes. Of his tapes.

Not legally, Tom reminded her.

Legal subtleties were not William Kroller's forte, she reminded him.

Billie could have killed Doran. But not Nielsen.

That would have had to have been dear ol' dad with a few details borrowed from the late Stephen Russell.

They didn't watch Robin's tape. Or Leslie's. Or B.'s. Nancy Rowe's, they watched. And learned nothing new. And then they watched the fourth video, feeling certain that they would learn something. And they did. That most psychotherapy sessions were boring. Like reruns of *Bewitched.* Only worse.

At eleven forty-five he left. He wanted to go home and shower and change. He'd be back later.

He ought to leave some clothes here.

He'd think about that.

"Be gentle with her. She is fragile and frightened."

"I will be," he promised.

She closed the door behind him. They had not kissed each other.

Chapter
XX

Tom knew a lot of people for whom the name Maxwell Street conjured up memories of a bygone era. To Tom it was not ripe with nostalgia. Perhaps he was too young for that. He knew that it had once been a flourishing street market crowded with immigrant vendors and shopkeepers. Jewish and Italian. And all of that bustling activity centered at Halsted and Maxwell. But that era had long since passed and the area had been downtrodden and seedy for as long as he could remember. Now it would need major renewal to reach back up to the level of mere seediness.

He parked in front of a boarded up hot dog stand across the street from the Mexican dump. No wonder he had not remembered its name. It had no name. Just a big handpainted yellow sign saying TACOS in large red letters. The storefront was directly under a streetlight. One of its windows had been replaced by wooden boards, the other had been painted over, several times, in different shades of yellow. The door of the dump was also painted in various hues of dirty yellow. Fortunately, most of the peeling paint work was covered with sheets of paper. As he approached, Tom could make out the words on some of them, the ones that were not too weatherbeaten or torn. One was the announcement of the opening of a soup kitchen down the block. That had happened in November. Which November was not obvious. One was about a church bazaar. That one was written in Spanish. The bazaar was to be held in January. Of 1993. Not bad. There was an announcement of a missing cat. Part of it was also missing. Were they looking for the cat? Had they found it? Or were they hoping to lose it?

Tom opened the door, trying not to dislodge any of the front-page news. It was darker inside than it had been on the street. The illumination from the streetlight could not penetrate either the wooden boarding or the layers of yellow paint.

Or the smoke. It gathered like the remnants of the Great Chicago Fire. He couldn't remember the last time he'd seen this much smoke without seeing a fire engine. Needless to say, the owners had never set aside an area for nonsmokers. Did they know about the city ordinance? About any city ordinance?

There were seven tables in the joint. Three of them were occupied. One by a couple. Two by unaccompanied women. The couple had to be Methuselah and his wife. He'd never realized that anyone could look that old and be living outside a nursing home. And she looked to be a decade older. There was not a tooth between the two of them. Nor a denture. They stared at one another, oblivious of their surroundings, their mouths half open. The only motion either of them made was the all but continuous pursing of her lips. And an occasional darting movement of her tongue. She looked like some gross parody of a cheap hooker. A class of individual well-known to this joint.

He'd been a cop too long. Everyone looked seedy to him. All women were hustlers. Especially if they sat in restaurants all alone. Hell, Dennie must eat out alone at times. The men in places like this were their pimps. Or potential johns. Or pushers. Or both. Or pickpockets. Thank god this wasn't Belfast. He didn't have to suspect people of being terrorists. Just ordinary, decent criminals. His eyes were acclimating to the smoke. And the darkness. The darkness was easier. There were women who weren't hookers. And men who weren't pimps. Or con artists. Or pushers. Or johns. Even at the corner of Halsted and Maxwell. He had to stop assuming the worst of everyone.

But not of those two women sitting alone at their tables. Like twins. Each was facing the door. Both were in their early twenties, going on forty. Each had a cigarette in her hand. And a single half-consumed drink on the otherwise empty table in front of her. And wore a sweater that was too tight and cut too low and revealed too much of unbrassiered breasts. Silicone? he wondered. Hadn't they heard that implants might be unhealthy? The least of their worries. They both sat with their knees crossed. Thighs showing. It was reassuring to know that his suspicions were sometimes justified.

And as he looked at the first one, her full red lips parted, the tip of her tongue darted out and then slowly wet her lips. Coyly. First the top lip from right to left, then the lower lip from left to right. Then the lips pursed into a kiss just for him and she smiled. A parody of a parody.

Goddamn hookers.

The second followed the same routine, somehow managing to push her bosom up at him at the same time. She looked more like a parody of some old lady who could no longer control her mouth movements. He owed Mrs. Methuselah an apology.

But not the two hookers. Why weren't they out hustling on the streets where they belonged? Because it was one o'clock in the morning. And it was only ten degrees out there. Not counting the wind chill. Wind chill was not good for business.

There were three men huddled together at one end of the counter. They were arguing loudly in Spanish. One man was sitting alone at the middle of the counter, smoking a cigarette and watching the two women. Obviously his stable.

There were four booths toward the back, opposite the far end of the counter. Where there was almost no light at all. Only darkness. And a fog of smoke. As dense as any London fog could ever have been.

Was that where the hookers took the johns on such a cold night? Why not? Methuselah wouldn't notice. Nor his wife. Nor anyone else. Except their pimp. He was there to keep score and collect the dough. Not to watch.

Tom walked back toward the booths. There was a figure in the last booth. A hooker? Plying her trade. No, the head was erect. Maybe there was another head hidden from view. No. The erect head belonged to a woman. She was wearing a hooded sweat shirt, with the hood up. And a muffler covering her neck and jaw. Above it was a half-smoked cigarette, still burning. Its trail of smoke didn't make the atmosphere any thicker. One cigarette couldn't do that. It also supplied the only source of light.

He could barely see the face as he sat down opposite her. What he could see seemed familiar, peeping out from behind the hood, the muffler, the cigarette, and the dark glasses.

"Tom Ward, I presume," she rasped at him. "I know I shouldn't smoke these things," she said, taking another full drag. The ring of illumination from the cigarette highlighted her face. He could see the black-and-blue mark below her right eye. Someone had hit her. Once. No, more than once. There were other marks. Older. "But the air in here is so bad, it's probably healthier to smoke a filtered cigarette than it is to take a deep breath."

"Beth?" he said.

"Who were you expecting, the Queen of Sheba? Or one of those queens up front?"

"Queens?"

"I'd bet they're both men. Or were at one time, but we didn't come here to discuss the quaint sexual proclivities of Chicago's young adults. Just mine."

She crushed out the cigarette and the features of her face disappeared entirely from his view.

"Should I get us something to eat?" he asked.

"We're not here to eat."

That was true.

"And the food in this place is not for eating."

"You've been here before?"

"With Mike."

"Why are you leaving Mike?"

"What are you, Miss Lonelyhearts?" she asked.

Not Ann Landers. Nathaniel West. Dennie had said that she was the literary one, the English major.

"Well, it isn't because I was born without a nose. Although if they open that kitchen door again, we'll both wish we had been."

Tom sat back. He too had read his Nathaniel West. Tom was used to being in charge. So was she. There was no reason to make it into a confrontation. Dennie wouldn't like that. Dennie. That was why Beth didn't want her to see her? She didn't want Dennie to see her battered face.

The face of a battered woman.

How?

By whom?

By the same guy who had mugged Dennie? Why not? Then why be ashamed? There was no shame in being mugged. That was one of the ordinary decent crimes.

"I meant to kill him."

"Meant?"

"In the same way that Achilles meant to kill Hector. In a rage. That's the subtitle of *The Iliad.* Did you know that?"

He didn't.

"The Rage of Achilles," she chuckled once. It was a chuckle reminiscent of Bela Lugosi at his eeriest. She was not someone to enrage for the fun of it. "Some translators use the word 'wrath.' 'The Wrath of Achilles.' I prefer 'rage.' 'The Rage of Achilles.' More balls. Leave 'wrath' to the grapes."

"We'd been studying together in the library. He called it a study date. I called it studying. I was working on Chaucer. In the original. Not in some modern translation. He was studying whatever it is that chemistry majors study. Can't be very interesting. It got late. The library closed. We went back to my apartment for coffee. I put on the coffee. I took off my sweats. I guess I should have remembered that all I had on was a thin cotton T-shirt."

She stopped. "Some coffee," she said. "I'd like some coffee."

Tom got up and went to the counter. He stood there for a moment and then a young, swarthy Hispanic came out of the kitchen. The odor was all Beth had suggested it would be. Both from the kitchen and from the hired help. Too bad there wasn't more smoke in the air.

"Señor?"

"Two coffees."

The young man wiped his hands on his dirty white apron, undoubtedly getting both dirtier in the process and walked over to the coffeepot. Tom looked around. One of the women was gone.

Was she a woman? Or a man? Or. . . ? That gave new meaning to the old phrase *let the buyer beware.*

The man put the two coffees on the counter. Tom put some cream in one and left the other one black. He could drink it either way. He grabbed a handful of sugars and picked up the two cups.

There was a man in the first booth. With one of the . . . let the buyer beware. Beth took the one without cream and used no sugar.

"He got turned on, I guess. I let him kiss me. And we fooled around a bit."

"Fooled around?" That could cover a lot of territory. Take it easy. Let her tell it her way.

Her voice was less forceful now. Less raspy. Almost pensive. "I didn't mind when he took my shirt off. It was kind of fun. He was a lot bigger than I was. And stronger. I wasn't into fitness then. Hell, I was probably in worse shape than Dennie is now. If you can believe that."

He protested. He thought Dennie was in great shape.

"For the shape she's in," Beth commented.

"He grabbed my head. His pants were open. He tried to force me. . . ."

"I get the picture."

"I finally broke away. I ran into the kitchen. And picked out the biggest knife."

She hadn't just grabbed the first one. She'd taken the biggest one. Still, it was hard to call that premeditation. Meditation in media res.

"He came after me. I lunged at him. I wanted to skewer him. En brochette. Right through his heart. I slipped and got him in the thigh. He thought I wanted to castrate him. I didn't. It wasn't the fault of his balls. It was his fault. I wanted to kill him."

The Rage of Elizabeth. Such rage. Beyond normal. Or was it?

Why did she have such a degree of rage? Was Doran right about such rage? Such anger? He had told Leslie that her anger wasn't anger toward her assailant. But rage directed at someone else. The real culprit. Rage like that came from the depth of the soul.

Was that also true of Beth? Of Beth's rage? Of the rage of Dennie's own sister? Her two sisters? Her sister who was two sisters? Multiple personalities.

Why? What had happened to Beth? What had caused her to become two people? It hadn't just evolved. Things like that didn't just happen. Not in the best of families.

What had happened to Jessie?

That, he guessed, would be the best approach. "What happened to Jessie?" he asked Beth, all but taking the bull by the horns.

"I no longer needed her."

"I thought she'd been a patient of Roger Nielsen."

"I was his patient," she corrected him.

"And he helped you?"

"He did. I became stronger. More me. I began to understand that she had become irrelevant. I didn't need her. She didn't need me. We were no longer each other."

"How? Why?"

"She had her life with Sean. I had mine with Mike. Mike won. She was better for us. I had Mike. I didn't need her anymore."

It was beginning to make sense to him.

"Love can do that. Not passion. Not lust. That's what Sean gave to Jessie. Passion. And he was good at it. But love is what matters. Mike loved me. Dear Sean. He told Jessica that he loved her. Maybe in a way he did. But what Sean loves is politics. Manipulating people. And their lives. Strutting into a courtroom and winning.

"Not holding me when we went to sleep, just to hold me. I needed to be held. And not just a prelude to a hump. What he wanted was what's going on in that booth."

She turned to him. "Do you love Dennie?"

"Yes, I really do."

"What would you do for her? To keep her?"

"Anything."

"I didn't kill John Doran. He was already dead when I got there. I was there. In the mall. In a car in the lot. I'd rented it from A.C. A real beater. Doran's last client, that black prostitute, she left at ten. I was waiting for him to leave. I had the keys. Then somebody else went in."

"Who?"

"It was a patient he'd seen earlier. A guy."

"Billie Kroller!"

"Yes. He was in there for half an hour. Maybe less. Then he left. I waited another half hour and then went in. Doran was dead. I made that tape. I left. I was in there for all of fifteen minutes."

"I saw the video."

"I figured you did. Dennie is not one to hide things from somebody she loves. She never has been. She is what she is. The best. The best sister. Don't mistreat her."

That didn't sound like a threat. But had it been one? Veiled but nonetheless real. Avoid the Rage of Elizabeth?

"Did you leave those tapes out?"

"Yes."

"Why?"

"I panicked. I saw a squad car drive through the parking area and I got terrified. I had tried to kill someone once. With a butcher knife. Who'd believe me? A dike who hated men. I fled."

"Did anyone see you leave?"

"I don't know. Why?"

"Did you lock the door behind you?"

"Yes."

"If someone saw you leave, then they knew you had the keys."

"I thought someone saw me go in. I had that feeling."

"Who?"

"I don't know. Kroller maybe."

"Or maybe not. Maybe his old man. One of his minions." Tom thought for a moment. "Were you mugged?"

"Yes."

"Did the mugger take anything?"

"My keys," she said.

Tom outlined his theory. Kroller's goons had been staking out Doran's place. To destroy his records.

"Of Billie Kroller?"

"No, of Leslie English. And they saw you go in."

"With a key."

"Right. So they mugged you but didn't get the right key," Tom concluded. "You'd given it to Dennie. So they got it from her."

"Poor Dennie. That was all my fault."

It was all making sense. Once they got the keys from Dennie, they went into Doran's office. "And couldn't figure out which tape was which. I couldn't. Except for the four new ones," he added.

"Which Dennie took but they didn't know that. And. . . ."

"That wasn't what they were after. They wanted all of Leslie's records."

"So they burned the place down," she guessed.

"And destroyed all of Leslie's records," Tom finished.

It made sense to both of them.

"I didn't kill anybody," she said. "I had no reason to. God knows I could have. But why should I have? I didn't know him. I'd never met Doran. Except as a patient. Once. I had no reason."

"Billie Kroller did."

"He did? Are you certain?" she asked.

He'd forgotten. She hadn't seen those tapes. Only he and Dennie had. "The taping. He figured out he was being taped," Tom said, and then described what they had seen. "So Billie must have killed him."

"Why didn't he take the tapes?"

"Maybe he panicked, like you did."

"He looked frightened," she said.

"But who killed Roger Nielsen?" he asked her.

She had no idea. It hadn't been her. Or Dennie. Or Jessie.

There was no Jessie, he reminded her. Tom got up to get more coffee for both of them. The other booth was now unoccupied. The two women, or whatever, were both at their respective tables. Neither was any the worse for wear. Tom wasn't even sure which one hadn't been there when he'd gotten the coffee the first time. Did it make any difference? Probably not. Any pair of lips in a dark booth would do.

"Señor?"

"Two coffees."

This time he did not even bother to wipe his hands on his apron. All things considered, Tom didn't mind. He didn't put cream in either of the coffees. Nor pick up any sugar.

Beth thanked him and warmed her hands on the mug before drinking any of the coffee. She didn't make a face this time. "It grows on you," she said.

"Like a fungus," he replied.

"What if Billie knew his dad's plans? That his dad was going to send in someone to destroy Leslie's records."

"Only they were tapes."

"Tapes that only John Doran could locate," Beth said. "What would he do?"

"I'm not sure."

"Leave them all there. And let his old man destroy them all. That way the joke was on his old man. In a way."

She could be right. She had to be. So who killed Nielsen?

"One of Kroller's goons," Beth said.

"Why the witchcraft rigamarole?"

"Witchcraft?"

"Satanic ritual, whatever."

What was he talking about?

She wouldn't know, he realized. It hadn't been on the news. Only the police knew. And Dennie. Dennie, not Beth. He described the murder scene to her.

"Brilliant. The perfect way to hide a professional hit."

"You could be right."

"I am. I have to be."

"Why are you leaving Mike?"

She touched her cheek gingerly. "Mike has a temper sometimes. And she gets jealous. For no reason. Of men. I can't believe it."

"I'm sorry," Tom said.

"So do I. Have a temper, that is. But I don't just hit. I lose control. I don't ever want to hurt anyone again. Especially not Mike."

"What will you do?"

"Jessie had some friends in Boston."

"Beth. You're not going to. . . ?"

"No. Jessie isn't coming back. Ever. That's all gone. That's over. But her friends can help me. That's what friends are for. Friends and family. One of them is a big-shot lawyer. I'll have Dennie sell my place. I'll be okay. And then maybe when I don't need Mike anymore, I'll come back."

"Tom, give me an hour. I want to say goodbye to Dennie. Give us an hour."

"How did you know I was going back to her place?"

"I was just hoping you were."

"I was. I am." He looked at his watch. It was just before two. "I'll get there at three thirty. Meanwhile I'll just sit here and watch the local entertainment. Maybe I'll keep score."

Beth got up from the both. "Bet on the one on the right. Bigger implants."

He hadn't noticed.

By three twenty, the score was three to one. The one on the right had won.

✳✳✳✳

Tom arrived at three thirty on the dot. Dennie was waiting at the door, wearing her thin silken robe and nothing else. She all but jumped all over him.

"I want you," she said. "Now."

"I want to see that tape. Beth's tape."

"Why?"

"Because she killed John Doran."

Chapter
XXI

"What did Beth tell you?" Dennie demanded.

"Wasn't she here?" Tom countered. "She said she was coming here. Where is she?"

"I don't know." That was one habit she'd have to get him to give up. Questions required answers, not counterquestions. "She has not been here once since this mess started, since we met. She didn't come home tonight. She was with you. She didn't even want me to be there." The cold air was creeping in from the even colder hallway. She felt a chill. All she was wearing was her thin silken robe. Wrong choice again.

"I'll bet." Tom tore off his coat, letting it drop on the floor just inside the door, looked around her large living room–office once, and then headed straight toward the kitchen. They both knew where he was going. Warrant or no warrant. Contiguous or not. Through the unlocked doorway into Beth's apartment. She closed the door to keep out the chill. It didn't help very much. The cold air wasn't the only cause of the chill.

"Tom Ward, stop this right now," she insisted. "Tell me what happened when you talked to Beth. My God, you've been gone for hours. I was so worried. About you. About both of you. You are the only two people in this world who really matter to me."

Tom stopped and turned to face her. His face softened. His jaw relaxed. "God, I love you."

Perhaps the silken robe hadn't been such a bad choice. "And I love you, too, but you know that." Did he? Did he know what he meant to her? How rarely she'd even felt like this? Anything like this?

"She asked me what I'd do for you," he told her. "For our love."

"What did you say to her?"

"I told her I'd do anything for you."

Dennie fought back a tear and said, "Tell me what my sister said to you." She was both relieved and more worried than ever. Beth must have said something to anger Tom so. To enrage this gentle being. Tom walked to her, kissed her once lightly on the forehead, ignoring her waiting half-opened mouth, took her

219

hand, and led her to her black leather couch. The two of them sat on the couch. The leather felt cold and uninviting to Dennie. Something was very, very wrong.

Tom told her precisely what had happened and what had been said at the Mexican dump, leaving out only the details of the two transsexual prostitutes. They, he thought, were irrelevant to his entire story. Tom told her that Beth had seen Billie Kroller go into Doran's office and then come back out about half an hour later. She had waited around for another half an hour and then gone into the office. She found Doran there. He was already dead. She had also told him about the other incident. And about Mike.

Dennie digested each word. She heard it all but she was lost. Lost and confused. He must have left something out. Some subtext. "But Beth told you she didn't kill him."

"She lied to me."

"How do you know that?"

"When she left, she asked for an hour to come here to see you. All by herself. I agreed to that hour. I sat there. For the first time I had a chance to just sit back and reflect on everything that's happened. The words. The evidence. The images."

"The images?"

"Yes, she showed us her guilt. In the video she made at Doran's that night."

"Beth's video?" Now Dennie was completely lost. She knew that video word for word. And it only had one image. Of a naked therapist with a knife jutting out of his back.

"I have to see it again, Dennie. To make sure. Maybe I'm wrong. I hope I'm wrong."

Dennie led him into her bedroom, put the video in her VCR, pushed POWER, and then pushed PLAY. At least he had had the good sense and the good taste not to tell her to play it again.

Tom held out his hand and Dennie gave him the remote control. He knew what he wanted her to see. And what he needed to see. Let him run the show. She'd sit back and watch. There was nothing on the videotape that she hadn't seen the first time. And the second time.

The TV came on and soon the image appeared. Once again the image on her TV screen was that of a man's backside. And once again the man was completely naked. The camera was still directed at the lower part of his spine. About four inches above the crease of his buttocks, which were no more enticing than they had been the first time. Or the second time. The camera remained centered about six inches below the wooden handle of the butcher knife that was sticking out of his back. The knife had not moved since last seen. It was still sticking out of the left side of John Doran's back, just to the left of his spine and just above the bottom of his rib cage. The same amount of red blood was collected at the base of the knife. There was still not much blood. The couch was still against the wall. And the angle of the knife was still about sixty degrees.

All in all, it was very much the way she remembered it, and just like before the man did not move. Nor did the camera. And there was no voice. No sound track. This time Dennie knew it wasn't the volume. So did Tom. He made no effort to increase the volume. He just waited, his gaze transfixed on the screen.

They both waited.

"Hi," Beth's voice said. She was winded, trying to catch her breath. "I'm back. I was just putting a fresh tape in Doran's set-up. In case you didn't recognize him. That's Doran. John Doran. Not exactly his best side. Just his most appropriate. His camera is fixed in the ceiling just like you thought. Right behind that little window. The actual recording goes on in a little alcove behind his desk. It's a very professional set-up. A fixed remote camera."

The image never varied. It never changed. No more than any of the oil paintings on her walls changed. This was equally immutable. But in a great painting, the more you looked, the more you saw. Would that happen to this image? It still just looked like Doran's naked back with that butcher knife sticking out of it. Beth began to speak again. "He was dead when I got here. I didn't kill him. But it sure looks like he was killed by a left-handed woman while they were making love. Would I let a fat slob like that make love to me?"

Another denial. What more did Tom want?

"Mike would kill me."

"She was probably right about that," Tom remarked.

Dennie said nothing.

"He was dead when I got here, with that knife sticking out of him and that little pool of dark red blood," she repeated. "I got in through the front door. I sort of borrowed his receptionist's keys. Not sort of. I did. To use the bathroom. And when I gave them back, she was a couple keys short."

At the mention of the keys, Dennie unconsciously felt the back of her head. The knot was still there and it was still tender. But at least the spinning was gone.

"She never uses her door keys. Doran gets here at nine and she comes in around eleven. She leaves at six. He sees patients . . . sorry, clients. If you can call them all clients. He sees them until eight or nine. Maybe later. She leaves around six. She still probably doesn't know I have her keys, which I don't. They are in the bag, taped to the bottom. There are two of them."

What was going on? What was he watching for? What was he seeing that she wasn't? Or hadn't? What was he hearing that she wasn't? Or hadn't? Or couldn't? She hated watching reruns. And this was no "Leave It to Beaver." This then was what she had seen before. And what she had heard before. Verbatim.

"Put them on your key ring."

She had done that. And look at what that had gotten her. This was maddening.

"What am I supposed to be hearing?" Dennie asked.

"Not hearing. Seeing," Tom explained.

What? There was nothing to see but a body with a knife sticking out of it and some dark red blood. Not much at that. "I. . . ."

"Watch!"

"A search warrant for my apartment will include your apartment but not your person."

There had never been a search warrant. Or at least not one that had led to any search. Tom had not gotten into Beth's apartment. He'd gotten into hers. Into her. That sounded better.

"Contiguous. The two apartments are contiguous. That's the key word."

Words were not what mattered. It was the image. They were watching, not listening. Watch. Look. See. What?

"It looks like he was making love to a woman. A left-handed woman who stabbed him. In media res, so to speak. And I do mean *media.* And I am left-handed! And it is a butcher knife."

And, of course, the body hadn't moved. They so rarely did. No matter how hard you looked at them. Watch. See. Dennie only half heard the rest of Beth's voice. Beth's narration. Bits and snatches of it.

"Think about it. Recreate the scene. Remember things you've done. Movies you've seen. Books you've read. Your fantasies. Even you ought to be able to. . . ."

"I'll be okay. I won't be home for a while. So I'd appreciate it if you could call Mike for me."

And the image never changed. A body that never moved. A knife that never changed its angle. And a small pool of violet blood that didn't get any bigger. That didn't grow or spread. Even reruns of "MASH" had more blood than this. Even cricket matches had more action.

Watch, she kept reminding herself.

But watch what?

"I'll be in touch. Hasta la vesta."

Tom pushed STOP.

"She didn't kill him," Dennie said. "You heard her. You heard what I heard. You saw what I saw. He was already dead, Tom. Beth didn't kill him. She didn't. She couldn't have."

REWIND. The VCR whirred softly.

"What did she say?" he asked softly.

"That she didn't kill him!"

"Not on the tape. To me. Tonight."

"What? I wasn't there. How should I know?"

"I told you. I'll tell you again. She said that after Billie Kroller left Doran's office, she waited half an hour."

"After Billie Kroller had killed him."

"No, after Kroller left Doran's office."

"That's the same thing," she protested.

The tape was rewound.

"Not quite."

Tom pushed PLAY.

"And she said she was only in Doran's office for a total of fifteen minutes," Tom reminded her. "Watch."

"I'm watching."

The image on her TV screen was once again that of Doran's naked backside. The camera was focused just where it had always been, about four inches above the crease of his buttocks. And about six inches below the wooden handle of a butcher knife that was still sticking out of his back. The same knife that was still sticking out of his back. The same knife. At the same angle. In the same damn place. With the same damn red blood collected at the base of the knife. Paschkes were more fun. Even Warhols were more exciting. Even a Georgia O'Keeffe vaginal flower. . . . She'd never thought she'd say that.

The same amount of bright red blood. She was concentrating on the details. The parts. Not the whole.

"Look at the knife."

She was looking at it. What else was there to look at? Certainly not his fat buttocks.

"And the blood."

And the blood. The red blood that was collected at the base of the knife. It was still there and it was still red. Knives did that to people. They made them bleed. The blood that was already collected when Beth had started to film her video.

Why was it already there? Because Doran was already dead. *Post res.* And he didn't bleed anymore. The pool never got any bigger. She'd bet on that. She'd stake her life on it. Beth's life.

And why didn't it get any bigger? Because he was dead. And had been dead for some time. Long enough to have stopped bleeding. To have stopped oozing blood. Dead men don't bleed.

FAST FORWARD.

STOP.

PLAY.

"Look at the knife."

She did. It hadn't moved.

"And the blood."

It was still there. No more. No less. She was right. Doran wasn't bleeding. Not an ooze. Tom was wrong. Whatever he had thought he'd seen wasn't there to be seen. The killer was John Johnston. Billie Kroller. One of them. Whichever one didn't matter. It hadn't been Beth. And they could prove it. With Beth's tape.

"He was dead when I got there, with that knife sticking out of him and that little pool of dark red blood," she repeated. "I got in through the front door. I sort of borrowed his receptionist's keys. Not sort of. I did. To use the bathroom. And when I gave them back, she was a couple keys short."

The small pool of dark red blood.

Tom was working furiously now. STOP

FAST FORWARD

PLAY

"I'll be in touch. Hasta la vesta."

Her Spanish had not gotten any better.

"The knife," he said. "Concentrate."

She was concentrating. As hard as she could. On the butcher knife.

"And the blood."

And the blood.

The blood at the base of the knife. John Doran's blood. The small pool of violaceous blood.

"There is no more blood," she shouted out. "No more blood. He wasn't bleeding. He'd stopped bleeding. Kroller had killed him. He was already dead. Just like Beth said." Triumphantly.

"Dead men don't bleed," was all he said.

She knew that. That was the point.

"That's not what you have to see."

"I don't see anything else," she said angrily. Was he blind? Only able to see what he wanted to see? Wearing blinders?

"Let's do it again," he said. "Just the blood this time. Just look at the blood."

She hated that blood.

STOP.

REWIND.

PLAY.

The small pool of dark red blood was just where it had been before. It looked no bigger. No damn different.

STOP.

FAST FORWARD.

PLAY.

The same pool of dark red blood.

STOP.

FAST FORWARD.

PLAY.

Of violaceous blood.

Blood was blood.

"Again?" he asked.

Again.

PLAY.

PLAY.

PLAY.

More blood.

Red blood.

Dark red blood.

Violet blood.

"She killed him," Dennie said. "Beth killed him."

"Yes, his blood coagulated while she was there making this video. While. During. Not before. It went from red to violet. From fresh to coagulated."

In media res.

"What are you going to do?" she asked.

"Arrest her. What choice do I have? Do you. . . ."

"Know where she is? No."

"I wasn't going to ask you that. I know where she's going. She told me. I was wondering if you'd mind if I lie down here for a couple of hours. I'm exhausted."

"Why aren't you calling in?"

"I'm off duty. And . . . she's your sister. I . . . I . . . have to give her a chance."

Tom fell back onto the bed. Dennie kissed him once lightly and said, "I'll sleep nextdoor."

He was already snoring.

She jabbed him once.

"What, I'm awake."

"Kiss me once and then take off your clothes and get under the covers."

Chapter
XXII

Tom could feel Dennie moving in the bed. That was one of the problems with trying to sleep at her place. Dennie's queen-sized bed was just too small for the two of them. She had said that she was going to sleep somewhere else. Probably at Beth's. Why hadn't she stayed there? Didn't she realize how tired he was? How drained? How pre-occupied? How distracted? How afraid that with all those distractions he just couldn't be sure he could do it? He couldn't go through that again. Not with her. Don't move, he willed. And don't touch me. She stopped moving. The bed had not been too small for their prior lovemaking. That had been just fine. Luckily, neither of them was into the acrobatic. Or the bizarre. It was sleeping for two that this bed was not designed for. His king-sized bed was much better for that. He'd tell her later. Much later, after he got some more sleep. Just a couple of hours more. Sunlight was already creeping in through the blinds. That meant that it was at least seven. He looked at her digital alarm clock. It confirmed his suspicion. It was barely after seven. Far too early to get up on a morning after you went to bed at five. Like early Sunday morning Mass after a late night on the town. He'd given up early Mass long, long ago. Almost as long ago as he'd given up late nights on the town.

Beth? What was he going to do about Beth? What choice did he have?

Beth was a murderer. She had killed John Doran. In cold blood. And then made that tape as if nothing had happened. She seemed so cool on that tape. Detached. Dissociated. Was that what dissociated meant? That she was out of touch with her emotions? With normal emotions? With normal feelings? Feelings like remorse. Much less guilt.

He would make his report and charge Beth with murder. And then let someone else try to find her and make the arrest. He didn't have to get any credit for this one. And he'd give her another couple of hours. She had only asked for one. He'd give her six. That left one more hour to sleep.

No, eight. He'd give her eight hours. That meant he had three more hours to sleep. That was much better.

She rolled toward him and put her head on his shoulder and pressed her body against his. She was naked. Dennie had told him that she always slept that way.

All he had on were his jockey shorts. Her body felt warm. And inviting. And those damn jockey shorts were getting too tight. Maybe he ought to take up nude sleeping.

Perhaps it wasn't quite as early as he thought it was. And perhaps a queen-sized bed did have its advantages. Perhaps Beth needed more than an eight hour headstart. Tom felt Dennie's softness against him. And her heat. She reached over and ever so gently pulled his face toward hers. She pressed her open mouth to his and pushed her tongue deeply past his lips. Her mouth tasted fresh and clean as if she had just brushed her teeth. She must have done that just before she crawled into bed. So damn sweet and fresh.

He sighed contentedly.

She sighed, but not out of contentment.

He reached across and began to rub his fingertips lightly over her breast. At almost the same moment, he felt her hand trail down across his chest, over his abdomen, and on down to his thighs, ignoring the growing contents of his shorts.

She emitted a deep groan and then her hand came to rest on him. Above the thin layer of white cotton. Why hadn't he taken them off before going to sleep?

He, too, emitted a single groan, just as deeply, but not as softly as he felt his flesh responding to her hand, becoming even more engorged. There were distinct advantages to her bed after all.

"Oh, God," he sighed. Sunday morning Mass had never been quite like this.

He was fully erect now. And her hand had worked its way under the cotton and had somehow extracted him. He could feel the fresh air below her hand and the slit of his shorts at the base of his sex. And he could feel that Dennie was no longer moving her hand. No motion at all. Neither up nor down. Not even squeezing. Just a tight grip that kept on holding him. Like some prize possession. To be kept in just that place. In just that position. The rest of her shifted. Moved. In a moment she was above him. Looking down at him. Her eyes fixed on his.

Her breasts dangled above his chest.

And her hips were suspended above him. And her hand was still holding him tightly.

Aiming him.

At her.

"I love you, Tom Ward," she whispered harshly, desperately.

"And I love you, Denise Cater," he said. "More than you know."

She pursed her lips and touched her right forefinger to them. It was not a time for speaking. For either of them.

Tom could feel her shifting her weight back toward him. She looked so beautiful. She was almost astride him now. Her hand was still firmly at the base of his sex. Holding him straight up in the air.

He felt her hair.

Her flesh.

Her warmth.

Her wetness.

Her heat.

Her snugness.

She sighed.

He groaned.

No one had ever been like this. Ever.

"You don't like to be on top, Dennie."

"I'm not Dennie. And I like to be on top," she cooed as he felt her wetness totally enveloping him right down to the base of his penis. He had never been that deeply into anyone. Never that totally enveloped.

He felt that he would push right into her womb. Right straight into her womb. He had never been in any woman quite like this. Right into her womb. Past her cervix. And into. . . .

She had not put in her diaphragm. Why not? She knew that. . . . This was her place. She had been in the bathroom. She'd brushed her teeth? She didn't want to get pregnant. Why hadn't she. . . ? Why?

"Not Dennie?!" he gasped.

"Of course not," she replied.

The toothpaste taste. That had been to eliminate the cigarette smoke. The cigarette flavor.

This was not Dennie.

Not the woman he loved.

It was. . . . "Beth!" he gagged, feeling the sides of her squeezing him more and more tightly, holding him inside her and massaging him in a gentle milking motion. Pulling more blood into him.

She nodded her head. And then began to move her entire body up and down on the fulcrum of his penis. Slowly at first. With a slight acceleration. Ever so slight. A very slight accelerando. This had to be a joke. It had to be Dennie.

It was her body.

It was her hair, dangling down on him.

Her breasts moving rhythmically above him. Swaying. So damn enticingly. The nipples lightly touching his lips. Asking to be sucked. Or licked. Or touched. He wanted to do all three. His tongue sprang out of his mouth, as if by reflex action. He tried to lift his hands to her breasts. He couldn't. He could not move them. She was holding them down. Immobile. His wrists were pinned to the bed. He was hers to do with as she pleased. And what was pleasing her was thrilling him.

Dennie.

Not Beth.

She had no black eye.

She was playing a game with him.

Play on.

And on.

Less and less slowly.

More and more deeply.

Dennie, he thought.

"Beth," she rasped.

Dennie.

Even more deeply.

Into Dennie's womb.

That womb he would someday impregnate. A child. Their child.

No diaphragm. No! It was not Dennie. It was her little sister. The woman who had killed John Doran in cold blood. And then been dissociated enough to make a videotape with the body. And now she was making love to him. Coldly. Dispassionately. Was she dissociated from him? Or from reality? She had to stop. To get off him.

"Stop," he requested. "Please stop."

She did not stop moving. Or squeezing. Or moaning. Or letting her breasts rub against his lips.

He wanted his excitement to stop growing. It wouldn't. It didn't.

He wanted her to go away. She didn't. She wasn't going away. She was breathing faster, deeper. More loudly.

"Stop," he said, "Please, Beth. Not like this. I love Dennie."

"If you love her, why are you fucking me?"

"I'm not."

"What do you call this?"

His hips were now following her rhythm. "Please don't do this."

"It's my going away present to you both. Something to remember me by. I am going away. You want me to. Dennie wants me to."

"Don't leave like this!"

"How else should I leave?" she panted at him. "It's perfect in its own way." Her breaths were short and choppy now. "You want me to leave, to go away. To never come back." Her breaths sounded almost like a succession of soft moans. "I'll never come back. But we'll come together first."

"I'm going to come soon," he gasped.

"And I'll come with you. With my sister's lover. Her beloved. My sister's husband-to-be."

"Aagh. . . ," he gasped. It was starting for him.

"So now whenever . . . aagh . . . you . . . you and Dennie . . . aagh, aagh . . . whenever you . . . you can think of . . . me."

He was now pushing upward against her hips. Not to get more deeply inside her. But to dislodge her. To push her off him. To be out of her. Out from under her. But instead it gave her something firmer to move against. And pushed him more deeply inside her.

He was about to come. He could no longer stop that. But he could stop this. This travesty. This sister act gone berserk. She was still holding his wrists in her clamp-like fists. Fists that resembled vices. She was so damn strong. All that weightlifting paid off.

Why was Beth doing this? Why? He continued to throw his hips violently.

"Aagh. . . ," she responded. "That's good. So deep."

Why? Revenge on that rapist? The one she tried to kill. Or someone else? Some other rapist. From her distant past?

She was dissociated. She had multiple personalities. From what?

He was getting there.

From something.

She was panting loudly now. And moaning. Rhythmically.

"You can be in . . . aagh . . . aagh . . . her and think of this . . . aagh . . . of me above you. Of my coming. Of . . . aagh . . . aagh. Of your climax."

And he was getting close. He didn't want to. He had to stop her. He couldn't. No. He could.

He had to.

How?

"I'm . . . I'm . . . almost," she panted at him. "Come with me . . . aagh. Tom, come inside me."

He felt a spasm enveloping his sex. And a weakening of the vice-like grips around his wrists. He jerked his right arm. It was free. He swung it as hard as he could. Up. At her. At this maniac.

"Aagh . . . I'm com. . . ."

His clenched fist cracked into her jaw.

Her head snapped back.

Then her eyes followed suit.

Her body jerked off him and tumbled to the right. Her shoulder bounced on the bed and she landed on the floor with a thud. He may not lift weights, but he had been a pretty good boxer in his youth.

"Aagh . . . ," he emitted through his gritted teeth and looked down as his discharge spilled out into the air and landed on the bedding.

"Shit."

It was over.

"Denise," he shouted, "where the hell are you?"

Tom got out of bed and leaned over Beth. She was unconscious. Her breathing was regular. Regular and shallow. There was no more panting.

Her pulse was also regular. And strong. He opened her yes. The pupils were not dilated.

She groaned. It was not a groan of pleasure.

She wasn't going anyplace. Tom put himself inside his shorts and pulled on his pants. He had to get Dennie. She'd know what they had to do.

Dennie! Where was she?

She wasn't in the living room. Or the kitchen. He crossed into Beth's apartment. She had to still be asleep in her sister's bed. "

"Dennie," he shouted.

No one answered.

The bed was mussed. And still warm. Where was she?

Out?

Running?

Only one thing was certain. She was not there. He walked back into Dennie's apartment. Was she safe? The thought sent a chill through him. Perhaps Beth had also given her sister a farewell present. A butcher knife. Nothing would surprise him. She was more than dissociated. She had killed before.

"Dennie," he shouted.

And no one answered.

Beth would know. He'd make her tell him. Where was Dennie? What had she done to her?

He raced back into Dennie's bedroom. And sat down on Dennie's bed. Beth was beginning to regain consciousness. "Beth," he said as firmly as he could. He'd be the good cop.

"Tom. Tom," she murmured.

"D. . . ." He stopped. "Beth."

"Tom, what happened?"

She was rubbing her jaw. "My jaw hurts. What happened?"

"I had to hit you."

"Why?"

"You wanted to make love to me."

"I did? Why? I remember now. I did. We made love. I came. You, you . . . hit me. Why?" She rubbed her jaw again.

She was still glassy-eyed, half dazed. It was the perfect time to strike.

"Beth," cautiously.

"Yes?" groggily.

"You killed John Doran."

"I killed John Doran," she repeated.

It was almost like watching one of John Doran's tapes. The one of Leslie English. Leslie English automatically responding to her therapist's every word. Following his every lead.

"With a butcher knife?" Tom went on.

"With a butcher knife," she repeated.

"Your own butcher knife."

"My own butcher knife," correcting the pronoun.

Did she own one? "Or was it Dennie's?"

"Dennie's."

"With Dennie's butcher knife?" he repeated.

"With Dennie's butcher knife," she repeated.

First degree. Premeditated. She'd gone there with the intent of killing him. She'd brought that knife with her. What choice did he have?

"Why?"

"Why?"

"Why did you kill him? Why did you kill John Doran?"

"He lied to Leslie. To his other patients."

"About what?"

Beth looked at Tom. Her eyes were less glazed over now. She was less groggy. Less dazed. She sat up and covered her breasts with her crossed arms, almost modestly. As if he had never seen her naked body before. Never felt those breasts. Never touched those nipples with his tongue.

Never placed his lips on those nipples.

He knew that he hadn't.

Her eyes were far less glazed. And her mind was far clearer. "About the witchcraft. He lied about that."

"The witchcraft?" he said following her lead.

"Doran made a mockery of it. He made it up. Leslie's mother had never been a witch. There were no witches. No coven. No abuse. Not of Leslie. Nor of any of his other patients."

"Other patients?"

"I was there the night before. At his office. Late. After he'd gone home."

"You had the keys."

"Yes. I watched his tapes. I couldn't figure out his system so I just picked a few. Randomly. And he tricked them all. He deceived them. He made up their stories. Their story. Always the same story. Of witches. And altars. And blood. And candles. And sex. Sexual abuse. It was not their story. It was his. HIS. John Doran's."

"I know," Tom reassured her. They had to get through this so he could find out what she had done to Dennie. "Ritual witchcraft does not exist."

She looked at him curiously. "Not in those patients of his," she agreed. "Not in the stories of his patients."

"So you killed him?"

"Yes. He lied. He made a mockery of it all. He . . . he . . . ." She passed out again.

"Damn." He had not asked her about Dennie. She was out cold. "Damn." Tom lifted her up and laid her down on the bed. Without bothering to cover her nakedness. He walked into the bathroom and held a washcloth under the cold water. He wrung it out and crossed back to the bed. She was beautiful. And resting as she was, she even managed a touch of innocence.

He began to wash her face with the cold damp cloth. This had to work. She had to wake up. She had to tell him about Dennie. Where was she? What had Beth done to her? Had she. . . ?

The makeup began to wash off.

"Beth," he said, "wake up."

She groaned.

The makeup was gone. The black eye was there. Beth's black eye. The black eye she had gotten from Mike. And the scrapes. And the other bruises. Where had they come from? From Mike? Why did women put up with such treatment? She looked as if she had been mugged. And she had! The bruises were all from the mugging. The mugging that had taken place outside his apartment.

"Dennie," he said, "wake up."

"Tom, what happened?"

"I hit you."

"Why?"

"You were making love to me."

She felt her face, her jaw. "Remind me not to do that ever again."

"It wasn't you. It was Beth. I hit Beth. She was on top of me. Making me make love to her. I hit her."

"Beth was here?"

"Sean had warned me. He told me. I just didn't hear what he said."

"What? What did Sean tell you?"

"That there was only one sister. I thought he meant that you had only one sister, but it's David who has only one sister. One! Not three of you. Or two, but one . . . I. . . ."

"You hit me," she complained.

"I hit Beth."

"Then why do I hurt?"

"Dennie, listen to me. She did it. She killed John Doran."

"Are you absolutely certain, Tom?"

"I know. She told me. She admitted it to me."

"What did she say? Tell me. I must know."

Tom told her.

"Beth killed him," Dennie admitted. "In a rage. He lied to his patients. He must have lied to her, too."

"What happened to her? To you, Dennie?"

"I don't know."

"She murdered him," he said.

"What are you going to do?"

"I don't know. I made a promise to Beth."

"To Beth?"

"She asked me what I would do for us. I told her I'd do anything."

"While you were screwing her?"

"Before, in that Mexican joint. You're jealous of her."

"I'd be jealous of any woman who climbed on top of you."

"Dennie, Beth has to go away."

"Like Jessica. Jessie went away when she was no longer needed. Beth is already gone. She knows I don't need her anymore."

"Already gone?"

"Yes. Beth is gone. I have no need for her any longer. She killed John Doran. I know she did. And I even know why. He created all those stories. I saw that. You saw it. With Leslie. And the others. He created their histories. So she killed him. She's gone. Beth's gone. And she knew she was going to disappear."

"Knew it?"

"She said goodbye to Mike. Mike knew that was a final farewell. That she was leaving her for good. That's why she made love to you."

"To me?"

"To my lover. To you. You are my lover. To you as my lover. Beth hated men." Hated. Not hates. Past tense. Not present. Hated.

"She had never made love to a man. Never. She made love to you to come back inside me."

Tom somehow understood.

"Beth is gone," she repeated.

"Like Jessie?" he wondered.

"No. Not like Jessie. She's dead. Beth is dead. Forever."

"Are you sure of that?"

"Yes."

"I love you," he said.

"You say that to all the Cater girls."

"No, just to you. Only you. You are the only one."

She sat up on the edge of the bed. A shiver shook her body. He pulled the blanket up around her shoulders.

Her hands were now cradling her head. She rocked back and forth. As she did, the blanket slipped off. Tom was standing in front of her. She reached back for the blanket. Her hand hit something wet. She drew it toward her face. She smelled it.

"Semen," she said.

"Coitus interruptus," he said. "I hate that."

"Will you think of Beth when you are inside me?"

"God, no! Never."

"I hope not," Dennie said softly.

"Go to the bathroom."

"I know. You hate coitus interruptus."

"No. I hate not being in you."

✳✳✳✳

"Will you marry me?" he asked.

"Do you always ask that question while you are making love?"

"I've only asked it once before," he said. "In a different lifetime. And," he added, "in one hell of a different way."

He waited for her answer. She looked so beautiful below him, her long blond hair strewn over her pillow. He stopped moving.

"Don't stop," she said.

"I need an answer."

"First things first," she said.

"Yes," he said. "First things first."

He moved more deeply inside her.

✳✳✳✳

They were both lying back on her bed, his head on the pillows, hers on his shoulder. They were both staring up at the ceiling. A little piece of glass would have been nice, she thought. A mirror. Even a videotape. No. That wasn't true. Instant replay was for other sports. A mirror.

"Will you marry me?" he asked.

"One condition," she said.

"What is that?" he asked, half afraid of her answer.

"You'll never leave me totally alone for more than a day or two, at the very most."

"Why?"

"I get scared when I'm alone and things . . . you know."

"I promise," he said.

"And I want to keep my own name."

"That's one condition?"

"That's it."

"Whatever you do will be wrong."

"What do you mean?"

"With your name. Dennie Cater. Or Dennie Ward."

"I meant Three Sisters Limited."

"That, too. Look at your literary precedents. Look at Scrooge. He left Morley's name up so he's a cheap SOB. A skinflint."

"Yes," she agreed.

"But not Sam Spade. Hammett would have none of that. Before the murderer was caught, before Archer's body was buried, Sam Spade had Archer's name removed. And that makes him cold-hearted. You can't win."

"So I can keep my own name? And it's still Three Sisters Limited?"

He nodded his agreement to both conditions.

"And remember one other thing. It was Beth who was the lit major."

He felt a sudden chill.

"Beth," she said.

"I didn't think about her . . . while, you know."

"I know you didn't, Tom."

"And I didn't propose to her."

"There's one more part to my condition," she said.

"One more! What's that?"

Dennie put a finger across his lips. "You will never again ask me an important question while we're making love."

"Is 'are you close?' a serious question?"

"Yes, but I hope you can tell that without asking."

He started to shift his weight.

She looked at him intently.

"I have to go to work," he said.

"Archer was killed by a woman. By Mary Astor, I think."

Her metaphor was mixed, but Tom knew what she was driving at.

"Sam Spade turned her in," she continued. "He sent her over for it. His partner had been killed. It was his job."

"And it's my job."

"So what is going to happen?"

"We're going to kill Beth."

Chapter
XXIII

Dennie and Tom drove to Glencoe in A.C.'s Corvette. Dennie now almost thought of that car as hers. Tom drove. He did not take the outer drive. They had no time for sightseeing. He took expressways direct from downtown Chicago to Glencoe. No stop signs. No red lights. No construction. Would wonders never cease? A few potholes. Those were to be expected. Until the Second Coming, at least. One of the Ellers greeted them. The one who had interrupted her in Doran's office.

Had he been the one who had bashed her on the head? He did have her keys. He had used them to let himself into Doran's. Had he been the black man on the roof? The black dude? The goon who had thrown the bucket down at her? Who had tried to make sure that she had kicked the bucket?

He smiled at her.

She could feel the spinning return. And the nausea. And the pounding. And her anger.

Tom took over. He showed his badge. They were here on official police business. Were the Krollers at home?

Yes. But the Krollers were not expecting him and his. . . .

"We're here and we are going to talk to them. Go get them. We'll wait inside."

Eller let them in and then he went upstairs. In a moment the Krollers appeared and in another moment the four of them were in the living room. The Krollers at home, entertaining. Tom and Dennie sat down on one of the plastic-covered couches. William Kroller took his place on what Dennie assumed was his usual chair. The same chair he had sat on the only other time she had been there. No sooner had he sat down than he pulled out a cigar and began to roll it between his thumb and finger and inhale its aroma without lighting it. Mrs. Kroller once again stood opposite him, at least twenty feet away from him. As if he might have a ten-foot pole. Or something else equally contagious.

The interior of the Krollers' house did not remind Dennie of a scene out of "Gone with the Wind" this time. It was no longer a misplaced version of Tara

237

using decor described by Margaret Mitchell. Or anything produced in Hollywood. Nothing that real. It was much more like a stage set for an opera. Some very dark opera. But more out of Kafka than Verdi. Hiding deeper and darker secrets. Not some medieval ritual. Down-to-earth twentieth-century mayhem and murder. These people had had her mugged. And then they had tried to kill her. It certainly wasn't their fault that they had failed. And they had killed Roger Nielsen. Billie wasn't around to thwart those plans.

No wonder their son had killed himself.

And their daughter was suing them.

"I assume this is not a condolence call," Kroller said.

"You assume correctly," Tom said, taking the lead.

"We've had too many of them. From people who didn't know Billie. And ones who didn't know me. Or either of us."

"We're sorry about your son," Dennie began.

"Really," Kroller said. "You hardly knew him."

"No, I didn't know him," she admitted. "Not very well."

"So let's just cut all the bull. What do you want, Lieutenant? I was told this was official police business." He was still rolling the cigar. And inhaling its aroma. He finally put it in his mouth, but still did not light it.

His wife had not moved nor said a word, but she was observing them all.

"We want your help," Tom said.

"You want my help? With what? You want to kill somebody?"

"As a matter of fact, that's exactly what we would like to have you do. We want you to have someone killed."

Kroller bit down hard on his unlit cigar. "I am not in that business," he growled through his clamped jaws.

"Since when?" Tom inquired.

"I'll ignore that remark," Kroller said, recovering his composure. "No one has ever connected me with a murder."

"It's my sister," she said. "Beth."

"Jesus, lady, you are some piece of work. And I thought my wife was cold."

"Tom, help me. Explain what we want," Dennie pleaded.

The three of them all looked at the police officer. All three needed to hear his explanation.

"Somebody killed John Doran," Tom started.

"Brilliant," Kroller said. "An outstanding example of brilliant police work. Another Sherlock Holmes. Who is this? V.I. Whatever-her-name?"

"Shut up, William," Mrs. Kroller said. "This man may have something of interest to offer us."

"Thank you, ma'am," he said politely. "As a matter of fact, I just might at that."

Mrs. Kroller moved into the room and sat down in a chair adjacent to the couch. William Kroller was now the odd man out, the one who was on the outside of the group. "Continue, young man."

Tom did just that. He presented their case step by step. Who had killed John Doran? One candidate was Billie Kroller. He had a motive.

"And what was that?" she inquired.

Tom explained. He did not give her all the sordid details, but just enough to make Billie's motive very clear to all present. Tom told them about Billie's discovery of the window and the camera.

Was Billie that afraid of betrayal? Or of discovery?

It was a rhetorical question. One only Billie could have answered.

"But he was not the only suspect, was he?" Mrs. Kroller added.

"No, ma'am. But he had both motive and opportunity," Tom answered.

It was, Dennie observed, like a parody of the classic whodunit. Hercule Poirot reviews the crime but without the suspects.

"But things didn't end there," Tom continued. "The tapes were still in Doran's office. Tapes you two wanted and needed."

"What tapes?" Kroller asked belligerently.

"The ones Leslie's lawyers kept us from viewing. Those included Billie's tapes. And the videos of the rest of Doran's patients. Including one very special patient, Leslie English. With Doran dead, his tapes of her became far more important to you. Very important. As possible evidence. Unimpeachable evidence. Evidence that could not be cross-examined."

"Maybe," Kroller admitted.

It was a routine even Dennie recognized. Not good cop–bad cop, but a variation. Good suspect–bad suspect. But who had the real power?

"The way I see it, Billie figured out about the tapes and somehow let it slip. And then one of you realized that there were tapes of Leslie's sessions. If he taped one patient, he probably taped them all."

"Not me," said Kroller.

Mrs. Kroller didn't bother to contradict him.

"You knew he had tapes of Leslie. So you had Eller mug Dennie to get the keys."

"How did we know she had the keys?" she asked. And in so doing answered Dennie's unasked question.

"Eller had seen her use them."

"Can you prove that?"

"Yes. That we can prove."

"And that he attacked her?"

"No, but that he used the keys." Tom went through that part of the story. Telling them about Dennie going into Doran's office and taking the four tapes, about her being interrupted by Eller.

Which Eller?

Did it matter?

In a court it would.

They all wanted to avoid ever going into a courtroom.

That they all agreed upon.

Then Eller had gone into Doran's and not found what he wanted.

Could that be proven?

It could. Beyond the benefit of a doubt. Only Doran knew which tapes were which. What to do?

Get rid of them all.

How?

Have Eller burn the place down.

Could that be proven?

The arson would be proven.

That Eller had done it?

That couldn't be proven. Yet.

"Not much of a case so far," Kroller announced to them all.

"He also tried to kill me," Dennie said.

"How?" Mrs. Kroller asked her.

"By pushing a cement bucket off a roof."

"Did you see him, young lady?"

"No, but Billie did."

"My son is dead," Kroller reminded them.

"Yes. And he'd tried to save me."

"Now why would he have done that," Mrs. Kroller asked, "if we were trying to kill you?"

It was a question that had been nagging Dennie for days, more persistently than the spinning. Perhaps. Maybe. . . . "Because . . . because you didn't want to kill me. You wanted to kill my sister, Beth. She'd been the one who'd been watching Doran's office. It was Beth who'd seen Billie there that night. Not me. Beth. That bucket was aimed at Beth."

"So what?" Kroller interjected.

Dennie now understood precisely what had transpired. The entire scenario now made sense to her. He was there to finger her. "We were standing there and I introduced myself to him. I told him my name. That I was Dennie Cater. Not Beth, Dennie. And then he pushed me out of the way.

"He saved my life," she told them.

"He fucked up. He always fucked up. That was him," Kroller contradicted her. A proud father to the bitter end.

"But you have no witnesses," his wife added. "Do you?"

"No," Dennie admitted.

"This is getting us no place. What's your deal?" Kroller demanded.

"We want you to kill Beth Cater."

"We don't kill people."

"There is one little catch," Tom added.

"What's that?"

"Beth doesn't exist."

It took some time for Tom to tell them what he wanted them to know. Not the psychiatric details. Just the outline of the story and the murder that would not be a murder.

"And why should we get involved? You've got nothing on us," Kroller reminded them.

"My husband does have a point there."

"We could spare you some embarrassment," Tom began. "And there is always the murder of Roger Nielsen."

"We had nothing to do with that one either."

"We could dig up something," Tom responded.

"Why would we have wanted to do any harm to Dr. Nielsen?" Mrs. Kroller inquired.

"He was going to be Leslie's expert witness," Dennie said.

"But he isn't now, young woman. I don't see what we have to gain."

"It's quite a coincidence that both of her expert witnesses were killed."

"Coincidences do happen," Kroller said.

It was pretty much a stalemate. "What if Leslie dropped her lawsuit?" Dennie asked, a step ahead of Tom.

"Would she?" Kroller asked.

"I think so," Dennie said, knowing full well that Leslie now had no case. Once Dennie told Sean what she knew, he'd be looking for a way out. She'd need a new lawyer, but she'd have no use for one unless she wanted to sue John Doran's estate for malpractice. Her case was as dead as her old therapist.

"I'd go for that," Kroller said. "What do I have to do?"

"Not so quickly," his wife said. "The suit has to be dismissed."

"Done," Dennie said.

"And Beth Cater murdered John Doran so that case is closed."

"Okay," Dennie replied.

"Officially?"

"Officially," Tom said.

"And one more thing," the older woman said.

"What's that?" Tom asked.

"Dr. Nielsen. She also killed him. And that case is also closed."

"Officially closed," Tom said. "Two solved murders."

✳✳✳✳

The plan was quickly worked out. The police had Beth's fingerprints from when she had been booked on that knifing charge. That was very helpful. They pulled the 'vette into the garage and emptied the trunk. Tom cut Dennie's wrist very superficially. Dennie spread her blood around the trunk of the car. Leaving several fingerprints inside the trunk. In her own blood. Bloody fingerprints that would match those in Beth Cater's police record.

The first step was completed. One of the Ellers would clean out the car. No other prints would remain. And then he'd park the car at O'Hare. And leave it there.

"But it's A.C.'s," Dennie protested.

"A.C. works for me," Kroller laughed. "It's my car. Not his."

"Can't it be traced?" she asked.

"Are you kidding? Would I handle a car like that if it could be traced?"

She hadn't been. But understood just what he meant.

✳✳✳✳

Once they got back to her apartment, they dripped some of her blood on Beth's rug.

An hour later Dennie called 911 to report that her sister was missing.

Who was her sister?

"Beth Cater."

"Elizabeth Cater?"

"Elizabeth Cater," she confirmed.

Detective O'Rourke would be right over.

All in the family.

"I wonder who killed Roger Nielsen?" Tom mused, half to himself. "We'll probably never know."

"Beth."

"Officially."

"Actually."

"Why?"

"Because he had never believed her."

Chapter
XXIV

The wedding of Denise Cater of Three Sisters Limited, daughter of the late Donald Cater of D. Cater Construction, and Lieutenant Thomas Ward of the Chicago police department took place three days later. The ceremony was performed by the Chief Justice of the Illinois Supreme Court. The witnesses were Sean Keneally and a member of the Cook County Board of Commissioners. He was a cousin of the late Donald Cater. It still paid to have political connections. For Sean it brought a final closure to a part of his life that he wanted to leave behind him.

Brother David Cater was even there. He brought along his entire family and even participated in the ceremony. He gave away the bride. He was so happy to have his one sister back that he wasn't even sure that he wanted to give her away. Dennie didn't give him any choice. She had never looked lovelier, nor more at peace with herself and with the world. If only mom and dad could have been there to see her this happy and this secure. At least David and his wife and her two nephews were. The only thing that David objected to was the wine. Who ever heard of serving Pinot Grigio after a wedding? Why not champagne? Was it too expensive? No, the wine had been a present from the Krollers.

David also came bearing gifts. He had bought them two first-class round-trip tickets to Paris. And a reservation at the Hotel des Saints Pères for as long as they wanted to stay. Unfortunately, Tom only had one week of vacation.

The Krollers did not attend. They were still in mourning. They sent the wine and Leslie sent a bouquet of flowers. Mrs. Kroller also sent an envelope containing a paid reservation for dinner for two in Paris at a very exclusive and undoubtedly expensive restaurant in the place des Vosges. Dennie knew the place des Vosges. She had walked through there the one time she had been in Paris. But she did not recognize the name of the restaurant.

Three stars, David told her. In the Michelin. She knew what that meant. Tom didn't. He struggled to survive on a policeman's salary. Three stars, he assumed, were better than one. A lot better, Dennie assured him. There were some things that he had to learn.

✳✳✳✳

The next day they took off from O'Hare on American Airlines. They flew direct to Orly airport. Orly was much closer to the Left Bank than DeGaulle. It saved them an hour's long ride in a Paris taxi and got them to their hotel one hour earlier. Being newlyweds, they put that hour to good use.

That same day the police, acting on a tip, opened the trunk of a red Corvette that had been parked at O'Hare for the better part of a week. No one was sure quite how long. The parking receipt wasn't in the car. Nor was much else. No papers. No crumbs. No obvious evidence of human presence. Until they opened the trunk and found traces of what appeared to be human blood.

✳✳✳✳

To start their first full day in Paris, Tom took Dennie to a spot just two blocks from their hotel, on rue Jacob, just off rue des Saints Pères. "I come here whenever I visit Paris," he said. "This is where it all started," he said, pointing to a plaque. "On this spot in 1783, John Adams, John Jay, and Benjamin Franklin signed a treaty with the representatives of King George III recognizing the independence of the United States."

There was a small unimpressive plaque on the side of an unpretentious building. The plaque was about the same size as the glass window in the late John Doran's ceiling.

"How often have you been here? And with who?" she asked. She had a right to know.

"Just once."

"And with who?"

"Whom, not who."

"Cut the stalling."

"If you must know, I was alone. How about you?"

"So was I," she lied.

That, they agreed, was best. And hand in hand they started their day of official sightseeing. They acted exactly as if they were newlyweds seeing Paris for the first time through each other's eyes. And they were. They did all the tourist things. They took the funicular up to Montmartre and visited Sacre Coeur. On place du Tertre, they munched on crepes and pommes frites cooked on the street corner. They had an artist sketch them and walked down rue du Bac to get all those views that Utrillo painted so poorly. Just like real tourists. They spent the afternoon playing tourists at the Pompidou and oohed and aahed over the Picassos and the Braques and especially the later cubist works by Juan Gris. And the Giacomettis. Sculptures and oils. Especially his quiet, gray oil paintings of faces. The Wadsworth show they had seen together had opened less that two weeks earlier and was still running. They'd go to see it again when they got home. They wondered if Paul Richardson and his wife bought one.

"I'll bet she made him buy one with lots of words," Dennie said.

Tom hoped she was right.

They moved on to Matisse. And the surrealists. Then it was back to the hotel to play newlyweds. Parisian restaurants served dinner late. Late sounded just about right. They had dinner at the three star restaurant on the place des Vosges. The place des Vosges they liked. It had been one of the world's first slum clearance projects, built by Henri IV in the early 1600s to transform the Marais area from a slum into an elegant region. It had lost some of its elegance, but nothing the Chicago Housing Authority ever built looked this good after forty years. Much less four hundred.

The Victor Hugo Museum was closed long before they got there. That may have been an omen. All through dinner they kept reminding each other of the restaurant's three star rating. They both thought that it was a glorified tourist trap. And they couldn't even order the wine they wanted. There was not a single Pinot Grigio on the extensive wine list.

Would Montrachet do?

No, it wouldn't, but what choice did they have?

Montrachet it was.

From a good year?

The best—they weren't paying.

✳✳✳✳

The blood in the trunk of the red Corvette was identified as belonging to Elizabeth Cater. It matched the blood stain the police had found in her apartment. That was not a good prognostic sign for Elizabeth Cater. They couldn't tell her sister, Denise, but they did tell her brother and her lawyer. Her brother seemed far less concerned than her lawyer. She was the prime suspect in the murder of two Chicago psychotherapists, John Doran and Roger Nielsen. The latter had once been the Chairman of Psychiatry at Austin Flint and was very well respected in psychiatric circles around the world. Elizabeth Cater had once been his patient.

Very little was said about John Doran and his reputation. Fair was fair. And besides, the Freudians controlled the media.

With Tom Ward out of town, Michelle O'Rourke found herself in charge of putting together the pieces of the cases, much as she was trying to repair the pieces of her own shattered life. All she had to go on was what Tom had put into the file. She assumed that the file was complete. She also assumed that it contained everything that she needed to know. What it contained was everything that Tom and Dennie wanted her to know. The entire official truth. Mike remained unaware of Beth's true nature. For her, Beth had two identities. She was her lover and the apparent killer of two men.

The possibility of a satanic ritual was mentioned in the press release given out by the police. As was a description of how Roger Nielsen looked when he was found surrounded by a circle of black candles. With one white candle in his mouth. Mike, out of concern for Beth, had not wanted to give out that information. Tom, however, had left specific instructions as to what had to be said. This was part of the official file, along with his reports and notes, both of which clearly implicated the missing Beth Cater in both murders.

The media loved it. Witchcraft. A satanic cult. Instant headlines. Talk shows. Editorials. Feature articles. Witchcraft had its biggest revival in centuries. It was bigger than Salem had ever been. Dr. Heinrich Slatter, of the Jung Institute of Chicago, gave several interviews on the role of satanic ritual abuse in causing behavioral problems. It was bound to be good for business. If there was stock in Jungian analysis, this was the right time to buy. Too bad John Doran missed all that business.

A Dr. Kris Swensen was also interviewed and gave a one-liner to a reporter. She called satanic rituals "the UFOs of the nineties."

✳✳✳✳

By the next morning the fingerprints from the trunk of the Corvette had been matched up. It was Beth Cater who had been in the trunk of the car. The prints matched the ones the police had in their files. She had been arrested once on suspicion of assault with a deadly weapon. Those charges had been dropped. The prints also matched the ones from her apartment. It was a positive ID. The car had no identifying serial numbers and was untraceable. And all the prints had been wiped off. None of that was exactly a surprise.

Tom and Dennie went museuming once again. The Musée d'Orsay. The Impressionists. The post-Impressionists. Cézanne. Renoir. Monet. Manet. Pissarro. She loved Pissarro. The most underrated of them all. Van Gogh. Gauguin. She hated Gauguin. They agreed to disagree.

✳✳✳✳

Leslie's suit was dismissed with prejudice. That meant she could not refile it. That night Leslie had dinner with the Krollers for the first time in almost a year. William Kroller had hoped that it would be a start. After dinner Leslie cried and hugged William Kroller and called him "Dad." She had missed him. And her mother. She hadn't known he was sick. Why hadn't anyone told her? Could he forgive her?

He could. He had also missed her. But now they were together and that was what mattered. That night he sent a fax to Paris. "Buy yourselves a present. The sky's the limit. The three Krollers."

✳✳✳✳

The fax arrived while they were having breakfast in bed. Thankfully, the maid had been too polite to interrupt them. The sky sounded like a pretty good limit to them. They agreed on what they wanted and spent their next two days doing the galleries. The sky was the limit, after all. And on the second day they found what they wanted. Not at one of the fancy galleries on avenue Matignon, although they did see one Jean Dubuffet that tempted them. Similar to the one that they had seen at the Pompidou. Their sky was not that high.

They located their present at a place called Dorothea Speyer's Gallery. Neither of them had ever heard of it. And what they fell in love with was an oil painting by Chicagoan Ed Paschke, Tom's old friend. And Chicago's premier artist. It was an oil of two female heads, joined together, like perfectly formed Siamese twins. Two heads joined where two ears should have been. The background began at the top as red-orange and ended at the bottom as a dark red bordering on violet and was richly textured throughout.

And the two heads seemed to move over that surface. In and out of each other. Neither of them loved the painting but neither of them could stop looking at it.

They sent the bill to William Kroller. Dennie was relieved that he had not killed Doran. And even more relieved that he had never molested Leslie. "See, it isn't always the father," she said.

"It certainly wasn't yours," Tom replied.

"What do you mean?"

"The death of his first wife."

"That accident. I'd almost forgotten about that."

"I hadn't. We looked into it. It was an accident. She was driving up to Wisconsin on a rainy day. Her car was demolished by a big lumber truck. Owned by Seltman Lumber in Waukegan. It was an old truck with an even older driver. Slow reflexes, bad brakes, and a wet road. A bad combination. The driver was lucky he wasn't hurt seriously. Just another accident."

Accidents did happen. Even in her family.

That day they also bought a pin for Paul Richardson's wife. One that looked like it might have been designed by Niki de Saint Phalle. But wasn't. At the store next to the hotel.

✳✳✳✳

On the day they flew home the Chicago police department announced that two murder cases were officially declared closed. There would be no further investigation into the death of either John Doran or Dr. Roger Nielsen. Elizabeth Cater had killed them both. She had at one time been treated by both of them and had undoubtedly not been happy with the outcome. The police were also convinced that Ms. Cater was dead herself. They thought that she had been killed by some other member of the same satanic cult. The result was another avalanche of headlines. More stories in "The Enquirer." And more talk shows.

Heinrich Slatter and Kris Swensen confronted each other on the "Oprah Winfrey Show." The studio audience was the largest ever. If you counted all the multiple personalities that had been created through satanic ritual abuse, that is. More personalities than seats. And no one was left standing.

✳✳✳✳

On the afternoon they landed in Chicago Tom told his wife that he had to go in to the department for a couple of hours. He had to make certain that the two murder cases had been officially closed. That all the loose ends had been tied up. That Beth Cater was officially dead. As well as guilty of two charges of murder. There had to be no excuse for any further official inquires in the murder of John Doran, the murder of Roger Nielsen, or the absence or death of Beth Cater.

What about the murder of that Williams girl?

What about it?

"My God," Dennie gasped. "Her own father had abused her and then run over her and killed her."

Had she been abused? Probably. By her own father? That was unproven. And whatever had happened, it had happened many years ago. It would be impossible to prove. She had to let it go.

But what about Happy Felsch? She, too, had been. . . .

"Clumsy," Tom reminded her. "Clumsy." They had to let that go, too. There was nothing they could do. The world was not a perfect place. Justice was not their goal. Survival was. Her survival. Their survival. Tom hugged her. They kissed. She knew that he was right. He'd be back as soon as he could. Did she mind?

No, she had phone calls she had to make and she was tired. They'd spent a lot of time in bed, she reminded him, but not much time sleeping. Besides, it was already after midnight, Paris time.

First she called Leslie. She was not at her apartment. She tried Glencoe. Leslie was there. Leslie sounded quite happy. She was back with her family, living in Glencoe. She was seeing a new therapist. One that Kris Swensen had recommended.

Next Dennie called Sean. He was glad Denise was so happy, that her life had straightened out. He wished her the best. The cases had been officially closed. Beth's file, like her life, was now closed. Sean never once mentioned Jessica. Her absence hung over their conversation.

Dennie was tired by then. The jet lag and excitement caught up with her. No sooner had Dennie hung up than the light on Sean's phone began to blink and the phone began to buzz very softly. Sean did not see the blinking. He was looking out the window, watching a lone ship on Lake Michigan. It was a freighter. He couldn't make out what flag she was flying. The first freighter of early spring. Not from Paris, he was sure.

It buzzed again. He knew it would keep on buzzing until he picked it up.

"Keneally," he said.

"Mr. Keneally, there's a Ms. Cater on the phone."

He knew Elizabeth and Jessica were gone. They would never return. What had Dennie forgotten to say? "Put her on," he said.

He heard a click and then a voice, "Hi."

"Denise?"

"No."

"Not Elizabeth," he said in disbelief.

"No," she chuckled, "not Elizabeth. Elizabeth is dead. Or don't you read the newspapers? You were right."

"Jessica!"

"Yes. Jessica. I just remembered something."

"What was that?"

"Didn't dad own some lumber company or other? Up in Waukegan?"

"You have a great memory. He owned an outfit called Seltman Lumber. He never put his name on the papers, but he controlled it. Your brother still does. Why?"

"No specific reason. It's just a fact of life. By the way, I'm back in town."

"Back? For a visit? I. . . ."

"To stay. For as long as I'm needed."

❋❋❋❋

Beth Cater's body was never found. In cases of satanic ritual abuse there never is any physical evidence. But the police know all about that.

❋❋❋❋

Two weeks after Dennie Cater and Tom Ward returned from their honeymoon, a certain Robert Williams, of Glencoe, Illinois, was struck down by a hit-and-run driver while walking his dog in front of his own house. He was killed instantly. The hit-and-run car was an old beater. Apparently either the driver never saw Mr. Williams or the brakes failed because there had been no attempt to stop the car. The old car was found abandoned several blocks away from the Williams' house. The driver was never found. Robert Williams was survived by his wife and twin daughters. One of them was a medical student at Austin Flint Medical College in Chicago. He was also survived by his dog. That fact and a few others were left out of the death notices.

And ThenThere Was One
A Two Sisters Novel
by Harold L. Klawans

It is March of 1996. Dennie Cater and Tom Ward have been married for a year. It is their first anniversary, but Tom is not in Chicago to celebrate it with her. He is in the Middle East investigating a series of terrorist bombings that had taken place in Chicago over the previous few months. These had been traced to the Middle East and more specifically to a bloody, internecine squabble among several Arab terrorist groups. His absence does not bode well for Dennie. Alone, she feels deserted.

Her other half, Jessie Cater, emerges and the two parts of Dennie's personality enter into their own struggle for survival. Dennie becomes increasingly desperate. She fears that she is losing control. She needs help. And she finds it. In a hypnotherapist who is able to probe her mind for the root of her troubles. He realizes that her so-called multiple personalities are the residue of her past lifetimes and that her struggle with Jessie is not new. It is the continuation of unresolved traumatic events in another lifetime. But which one? And how can Dennie be helped? He is certain that she can; but only through reliving her past lives and resolving her past conflicts. Then and only then can she triumph as the sole surviving personality.

With the help of this therapist, Dennie undertakes a journey through her past, a past that spans centuries, lifetimes, and worlds. In the process she emerges into an unsuspected parallel life as a member of a terrorist cell whose assignment is to kill Tom Ward.